D0602176

BASIC
fitness on the ball

BASIC

fitness on the ball

Lorna Lee Malcolm

MQP

About the author

Lorna Lee Malcolm qualified as a solicitor, then entered the fitness industry in 1985. Currently the Fitness Director at the Reebok Sports Club, London, Lorna is the author of two previous books and was included in an industry "Top 10" published in a major British national newspaper. As a Reebok Master Trainer and Pure Energy Select Presenter, Lorna trains people all over the world, has appeared on television, and is frequently featured in magazine and newspaper articles.

This book is dedicated to my mother in law, Clarise, who has left this world and my niece Safiya, who has joined us.

Caution

If you are pregnant, have given birth in the last six weeks, or have a medical condition, such as high blood pressure, spinal problems, arthritis, or asthma, consult your medical practitioner or an experienced teacher before any exercise.

Published by MQ Publications Limited
12 The Ivories
6–8 Northampton Street
London N1 2HY
Tel: 020 7359 2244
Fax: 020 7359 1616
Email: mail@mqpublications.com
Website: www.mqpublications.com

Copyright © MQ Publications Limited 2004
Text © Lorna Lee Malcolm 2004

Editor: Abi Rowsell
Design: Balley Design Associates
Illustrations: Oxford Designers & Illustrators
Photography: Stuart Boreham

ISBN: 1-84072-498-6
1 3 5 7 9 0 8 6 4 2

All rights reserved. No part of this publication may be reproduced or transmitted in any form or by any means, electronic or mechanical, including photocopy, recording, or any information storage and retrieval system now known or to be invented without permission in writing from the publishers.

Printed in China

contents

foreword

Ask a group of people why they don't exercise, particularly now, when we know that regular exercise or physical activity is good for us, and you will get a number of different answers that will usually fall into a few common categories.

One of the things I often hear is that people don't exercise because they find it boring. In that instance, I would say the ball is definitely for you. It is different to so many of the traditional ways of exercising and it challenges the body on a variety of different levels all at the same time. In this book you will find different exercises for the same muscle group, different positions for similar exercises and a number of sequences you can follow that focus on different objectives so that you don't have to do the same exercises in the same way every time.

"Boring" can also be a state of mind. Don't think of it as a chore. Be positive about your exercise and the benefits you will get from it.

Lack of time is another common reason given for not exercising. With the ball you can exercise in the comfort and convenience of your own home and fit your exercise in to suit your day. Yes, you may still have to find that extra 30 minutes but you will if your health and well-being are important to you.

At least you won't have to travel to and from the gym, and spend time changing and showering afterward. You can do a session when you get up, showering afterward as part of your normal routine for getting ready for work, or do a session when you get home, in which case you are likely to be more relaxed about it and have a shower/bath afterward to aid relaxation and to make the whole experience part of the "personal time" you are investing in yourself. Set aside time in your diary for your sessions, just as though they are important appointments that you have with yourself. Commit to them and don't let yourself down but, if you just can't fit it in, don't stress about it. There is always another day.

The "I can't afford it" statement should definitely not come into consideration. Using a ball is one of the least expensive ways to get an effective and efficient workout. All you need is your ball, this book and a mat or towel that you will already have at home. Hand weights are featured in this book but they are not essential and should not deter you from starting. They can be a later investment or you could ask someone to buy them for you for your birthday or Christmas.

"It's too hard" is also an invalid answer. The exercises in this book come with "easy" or "moderate" ratings. There are also modifications given relative to position, repetitions and timing that should all help you start and progress the exercises in the best way for you.

So there it is. No excuses. Get started with a positive mental attitude and see what results you achieve. Remember that the results will be a reflection of your commitment and investment in exercising regularly and being more active generally. As well as working out with your ball, don't forget to do some cardiovascular exercise—just using stairs instead of the elevator, walking instead of using the car—all things that will make your lifestyle more active.

Have fun and enjoy.

Lorna Lee Malcolm

introduction to the ball

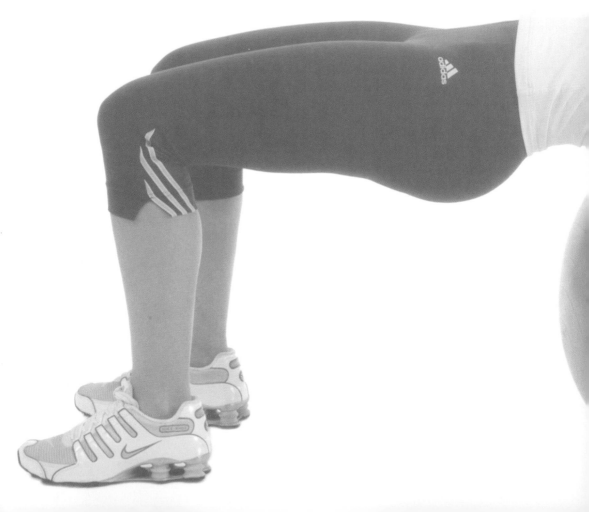

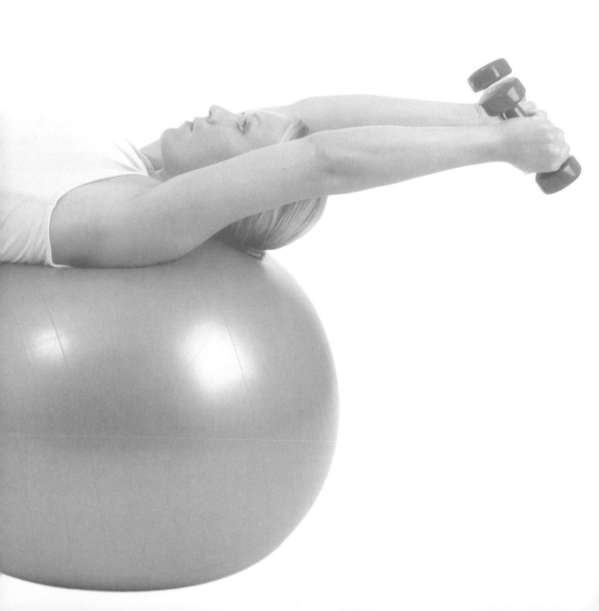

why use a ball?

Exercising with a ball is a fun, inexpensive but challenging way to work out and achieve real results—ball fans delight in feeling fitter and stronger and looking leaner. The ball itself is known by a variety of different names. You may hear it called a stability ball, fit ball, gym ball, resist-a-ball, physio ball, or Swiss ball to list a few. Whatever you call it, though, you can be confident that it has a long, distinguished, tried and tested pedigree. It comes to us from physiotherapy and rehabilitation clinics where it has been used for many years to assist in the treatment of spinal injuries, neurological disorders, and orthopedic problems.

Ball sizes

The balls come in a range of sizes and it is important to comfort and positioning that you work with a ball that is the appropriate diameter for you. The guideline is that when you are seated on the ball, your knees should be in line with your hips or just a touch higher and parallel to the floor.
The most common ball diameters are:

- 18 inches (45cm)
- 22 inches (55cm)   ■ 26 inches (65cm)

Be aware that the softer the ball, the easier the exercises will be as the body is able to sink more into the ball. The firmer the ball, the harder the exercises will be.

Care and Storage
You can store your ball inflated, as long as you top up the pressure if it starts feeling soft or is visibly deflating. A bicycle pump, compressor, or the pumps used in garages and bicycle shops can be used but always follow the manufacturer's instructions.

It is possible to inflate your ball so that it is firm but still remains quite small. The trick is to overinflate it and then let some air out.

Clean your ball with a damp cloth or mild soapy water. Store it in a cool, dry place and avoid excessive or intense heat, which can damage it.

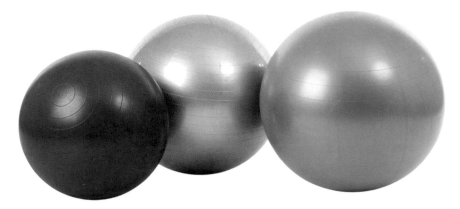

The ball has rolled into the health and fitness world in the past ten years and it is becoming a common piece of equipment, used in health clubs for personal training and, more recently, group exercise classes. It is also finding its way into homes and work places as people realize that the ball not only has exercise benefits but also is a great tool for addressing postural alignment and core stability weaknesses.

Muscle	Common name	Location in the body
Hamstrings	Hamstrings	Group of muscles at the back of the thigh
Gluteus maximus	Glutes	Large buttock muscles
Lattissimus dorsi	Lats	Muscle just under the shoulderblade
Abdominals	Abs	Four specific muscle groups in the torso
Quadratus lumborum	Quadratus lumborum	Muscle to the side of the torso; helps keep you upright
Quadriceps	Quads	Four muscles that make up the front of the thigh
Adductors	Inner thighs	Muscles of the inner thigh
Abductors	Outer thighs	Muscles of the outer thigh
Tibialis anterior	Shin	Muscles at the front of the lower leg
Rectus abdominus	Six pack	Most superficial of the abdominal group; runs down the front of the torso
Internal and external obliques	Obliques	Second and third sets of abdominals; run from the waist area toward the groin
Transverse abdominus	Transverse or T.A.	The deepest abdominal muscle; the one most concerned with core stabilization
External hip rotators	External hip rotators	Muscles around the side of the hip joint; enable the leg to turn outward
Hip flexors	Hip flexors	Muscles at the front of the hip joint
Rotator cuff	Shoulder rotators	Muscles within the shoulder joint that enable the arms to turn in and out

Main muscle groups (front of body)

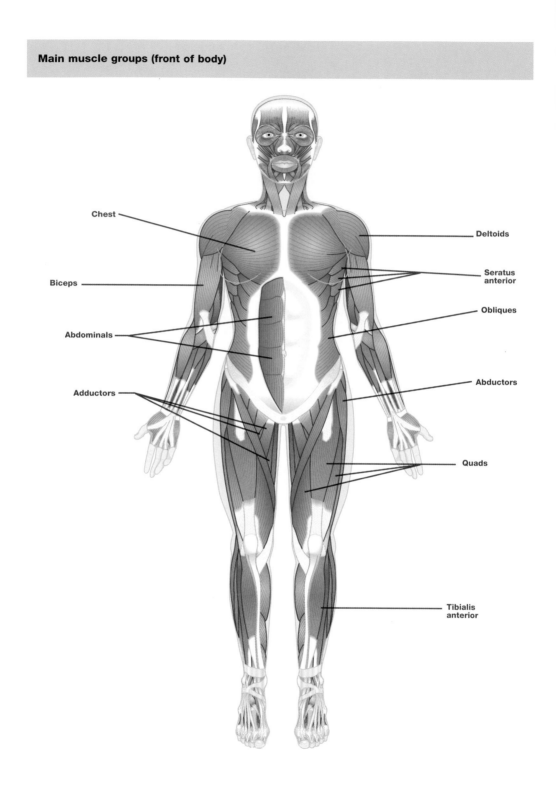

Chest

Deltoids

Seratus anterior

Biceps

Obliques

Abdominals

Abductors

Adductors

Quads

Tibialis anterior

Main muscle groups (back of body)

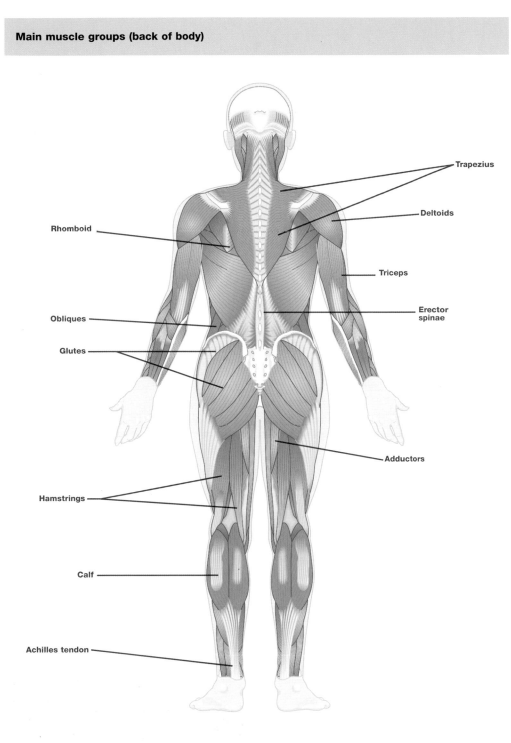

Trapezius

Deltoids

Rhomboid

Triceps

Erector
spinae

Obliques

Glutes

Adductors

Hamstrings

Calf

Achilles tendon

the benefits of stability ball training

Training with a stability ball has a number of benefits.

improved core strength and stabilization

Where exercises are done on or with an unstable, dynamic piece of equipment, there is more involvement of the core muscles of the torso, whether or not the limbs move.

The "core" of the body is foundational to all movement and activity as well as to balance, coordination, and stability, but for many years the core has been ignored in favor of:

- developing muscle for esthetic reasons, as with body building
- staying within very traditional modes of fitness and training
- working primarily on cardiovascular fitness because many people believe that only sweat equates to hard work.

Having a strong core is foundational to all of the above and translates back into all fitness and physical activity, strenuous or otherwise. Strength of the core affects posture and alignment, muscle balance, and muscle synergy. It can affect how you move or hold a position in a step or yoga class, how you carry the shopping, sit at your desk, or carry yourself as you walk. It affects everything the body does, be it still or moving.

Working with machines in the gym has not addressed the issue of core stability because people tend to rest into the back pads of the machines and rely on them for support rather than using their own muscles to support themselves as they carry out the exercise.

Until fairly recently in fitness programs, we essentially worked each muscle group separately. For example, we would do a

biceps exercise and then a triceps exercise, followed by hamstrings, glutes, and so on, going through our muscle list like a shopping list. We now know—from research and learning more about how the body functions—that muscles should also be worked in unison. For example, you should regularly train the abdominals and the back together, as doing so improves the working relationship they have with each other. We should always be conscious of what related muscles are doing.

As a result, most of the exercises in this book will have more than one benefit and work more than one muscle group at the same time. Most have an element of balance (and not just in a standing position) and all require focus on posture and alignment, which encompasses core stability and works toward gaining a stronger, leaner torso.

below> **Core stabilization in action.**

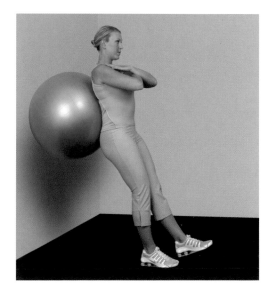

better range of movement

Working with the ball often allows a greater range of movement for the exercise because of how the body is placed. Being off the floor gives wider scope in exercise choice and influences how you do an exercise. The ball enables exercises to be done in a variety of different positions so that sometimes gravity assists the movement, sometimes gravity is neutralized, and at other times gravity resists the movement, making it harder.

External support with a stability challenge can still be obtained by placing the ball against a wall. You can also use the ball with your feet anchored against the wall. The ball allows for structured and natural progressions from easier to harder levels of the same exercise by manipulating body position and limb length (for example, a bent arm or leg is easier to lift than a straight arm or leg). Additional progressions are also possible through introducing external resistance—for example, by using handweights.

improved posture and alignment

Using the ball improves balance and coordination, posture, and alignment, and results in increased body awareness. Neutral alignment is good posture because "neutral" refers to the body being aligned in a way that is the least stressful to the skeleton, muscles, and the body's neural system. Bad posture is usually the result of muscle weakness and malfunction, muscle imbalance, and a lack of body awareness. Genetic factors may predispose some people toward bad posture (for example, if you are born with one leg longer than the other and you don't work on strengthening the resulting problem areas). However, bad posture is often caused by lifestyle—ways of working, sitting, and standing, leisure activities, gravity, and so on.

It is generally agreed that the better your posture, the better you function and the lower your risk of injury. Bad posture causes a lot more stress to the joints and muscles and small stress injuries that happen repeatedly and frequently over a long period of time, will cause aches and pains. This is a common cause of back pain.

Working on the ball requires postural muscles to be used all the time and so strengthens and improves the working relationship between all the muscles that contribute to good posture. The Standing chapter sets out "neutral" alignment and reminders to maintain it will be given in all subsequent chapters.

proprioreception and body awareness

Body awareness is not just about how the body is but also about where it is in space. Proprioreception is the body's ability to adapt to changes of position through sensors and receptors of the neural system. This system works joint by joint and muscle by muscle. If not challenged, it can become lazy and skills like balance and coordination can deteriorate as a result. The ball taxes this aspect of the body with every exercise and so should improve awareness of the body in space. It also ensures that the muscles around the joints stabilize when they should to protect the joints from injury. The ball can be used to improve strength and flexibility and can also be incorporated into a more cardiovascular application.

The joy of exercising with a stability ball is that as well as delivering all-round benefits, it turbo-charges the intensity of conventional moves, so that a workout that takes only 30 minutes to complete can yield serious results. Once you get started, you'll soon feel that fitness is, quite literally, a whole new ball game.

When we talk about the core, we are in part referring to an inner unit or cylinder within the torso area. If trained properly, the core muscles can make you stronger from the inside out. The pelvic floor muscles form the bottom of the cylinder and the diaphragm the top. The deep abdominal muscle—the transverse abdominus—makes up the front and part of the sides, and is attached to the back. The multifidus muscle that runs lengthwise along the spine makes up the rear section. These muscles stabilize the sacrum, or lower spine, as well as the joint where sacrum and pelvis meet.

The core is also supported by muscles close to the center of the body, such as the erector spinae, the quadratus lumborum and the internal obliques.

When all these muscles are activated at the same time, it is like wearing the sort of weight belt that bodybuilders use to help them with their training. Luckily for us, if the core is working as it should, it can make us move more efficiently and reduce neck tension and upper and lower backache.

In addition to the inner unit, other muscles contribute to core stability—the muscles of the bottom and hips, the other abdominals and lower back, and the muscles of the upper back and legs.

Traditional torso training consisted primarily of curls and sit-ups and concentrated on development of the "six pack." However, research now shows that we need to be working all the core muscles and regularly training them together.

To stabilize your core, you need to switch on your pelvic floor, abdominals, and back muscles simultaneously. To activate your pelvic floor muscles, imagine that you need to get into a pair of jeans that are a half size too small. The muscles should contract and draw up internally. Try to keep the activation as you draw your navel toward your spine. Your waist should feel at least half an inch (1.3cm) smaller and you should feel "tone" in the whole of the stomach area, from under your ribs to your pubic bone.

The trick is to train your body so the movement becomes automatic and your muscles can maintain it when your mind is on something else. The second step is to keep the activation and internal stabilty as you move, for although movement happens through the limbs, often that movement starts in the torso. The torso will always be involved because it links the upper and lower body.

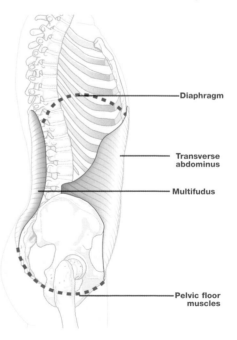

Diaphragm

Transverse abdominus

Multifudus

Pelvic floor muscles

exercising with the ball

Some enthusiasts can be seen sitting at their desks having swapped their regular office chair for a ball because it heightens awareness of sitting posture and encourages better alignment. This can help strengthen the back and the deep abdominals and reduce the incidence of lower back pain.

The ball has a dynamic nature in that it moves. It challenges balance and stabilization at the same time as the user works on strength and/or flexibility. This provides functional training where the body is worked as a unit (a whole) and different muscles are worked together, whereas traditionally we have worked each muscle or muscle group separately.

In most exercises there will be elements of strength required of some muscles and elements of flexibility required of others. There will be demands made on the mobility of a joint and the stability of a joint within the strength and stretching exercises. Some muscles hold while others move. These demands simply mimic the demands that are made on the body in daily life.

Think about the movement of picking up two shopping bags at the supermarket and carrying them to the boot of your car. There are some muscles responsible for the walking action, others working to stabilize the pelvis as that movement happens. Some upper body muscles are involved in carrying the weight of the shopping while others ensure that we don't put our back out or strain something as we carry the shopping and walk at the same time. Neck and back muscles work to hold our head in place so that we can see where we are going. It is always a concerted effort.

Part of the success in using a ball will come from mimicking that concerted effort by doing compound and integrated exercises that work different muscle groups at the same time and encourage the upper and lower body to work together. Another part of the success will come from developing and improving the skills to be able to control the body and the ball at the same time. The first step is to be able to get into and maintain the start position with good alignment. The second step is to execute the movement with control of the body and the ball. Additional progressions are included in some of the exercises.

below> **Concerted effort is required to hold this position.**

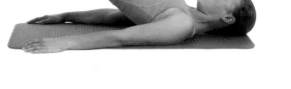

stretching

A range of stretches are included in this book. If you have not exercised or stretched for a while, passive stretching is probably a good way to start. "Passive" means "non-active" and these stretches are so labeled because no muscles are actively contracting in order for the stretch to occur. These types of stretches are usually also done "statically," where the position is held for a period of time.

Active stretches are those in which some muscles (usually the opposing muscle group) contract and work, while the stretching muscle group relaxes and lengthens. These stretches are often more intense and more challenging than those done passively.

You will see that the stretches are to be held for a number of breaths rather than a given time. The reason for the use of the breath to time a stretch is twofold. Firstly, it gives the mind something to focus on that is not complex or taxing and so should aid relaxation of mind and muscles. Secondly, it means that you don't have to keep your eye on a watch to check when 30 seconds have passed, which could create tension.

Stretching should not always be easy or comfortable. Often, to develop flexibility, the initial position or extent of the stretch should pull the muscle so that the stretch is on the edge of discomfort. As the muscle fibers lengthen, the discomfort should ease.

warm-up

Don't forget to warm your muscles up before starting as a way of preparing both muscles and joints for the work that is to come. If you feel tight in any area of the body or if you have been sitting for long periods, a short pre-workout stretch focusing on the muscles you are going to use and the muscles that seem tight can be included.

As well as including a full range of motion movements that use the large muscle groups of the legs and mobility movements for the upper body, your warm-up should contain an element of what you are going to do in the workout itself. Think of it as being like a practice run or a rehearsal at low intensity. The standing twists, lunges, moving hip hinge, and standing squats that are featured in the Standing chapter, and the pelvic tilts and single leg balance, described in the Seated chapter, could all be incorporated in a good warm-up sequence. These are exercises that will get the body moving, raise your body temperature a little, and activate the muscles that are about to work.

The warm-up is also meant to increase the heart rate so that warm blood gets pumped around the body faster. The result is that your muscles will be more pliable. Warming up also affects the synovial fluid of the joints, ensuring better lubrication, which then allows easier joint movement, a greater range of movement, and less risk of injury and soreness.

The warm-up also brings about an increase in neural impulses, which is particularly important for reducing any tendency to instability. And the metabolic rate and oxygen uptake increase as the body requires more oxygen to create energy to carry out the exercises.

Another part of the preparation will always be mental. This psychological aspect should not be overlooked as it will contribute to the heightened sense of body awareness and the ability to perform physically.

Remember also that age, ability, or fitness level, and the environment can all affect the amount of time you should spend warming up. Your warm-up should be longer if you are (relatively) older, not that fit, or if the environment is cold or cool.

If you are also performing any sort of cardiovascular activity, such as going for a run, rollerblading, or power walking, it is best to do your ball workout when your return. Then you will already be warm and your body will be well prepared.

For an example of a warm-up sequence, see pages 20–23.

cool-down

You would usually be advised to cool down after a workout. However, because this work-out is not cardiovascular, fast, or furious, but quite slow and controlled in its application, a specific cool-down is not necessary. Stretching, which is important to any kind of workout, can either be done at the end of, or interspersed during, the workout.

wind-down

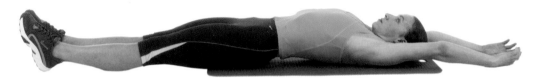

If you are doing your workout toward the end of the day, you may find it beneficial to finish your session with a "wind down" relaxation. Lie on your mat on the floor and stretch your arms above your head so that the backs of

your hands touch the floor. Imagine that one person is holding your wrists and another your ankles. Feel yourself grow at least half an inch (1cm). Hold for 3 to 5 deep breaths, then slowly release.

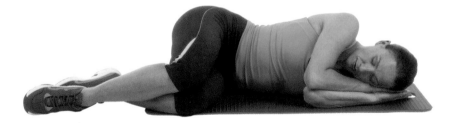

Now turn yourself onto your side and pull your knees up toward your chest so you are lying in a fetal position. Place one or both hands under your lower cheek or rest your head on a small pillow. Close your eyes and try to clear

your mind. If you cannot achieve this, try not to think about anything specific unless it assists your relaxation. You might like to listen to some soothing music to help you relax. Lie in this position until you feel ready to stand up.

get the body moving

Unless you have done some cardiovascular exercise before using your stability ball, try this example warm-up sequence. When you have finished you should be ready for a full workout.

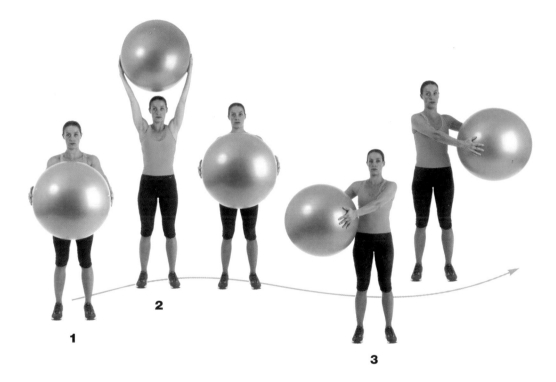

1 Stand with your feet hip-width apart with the ball held out in front of you. Set your posture and alignment as already described, and activate your core muscles.

2 Take a deep breath in and lift the ball over your head, keeping your arms straight and your torso strong and set. Avoid arching your lower back as you lift your arms overhead. Lower the ball as you breathe out. Repeat 8 times.

3 Hold the ball in front of you and twist your body from one side to the other, first keeping your hips facing forward and then allowing your hips to twist with the movement. Do 8 of both types of twist.

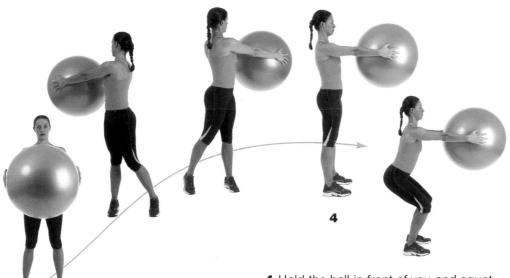

4 Hold the ball in front of you and squat back, as if there is a chair behind you that you are about to sit on but then you change your mind.

3

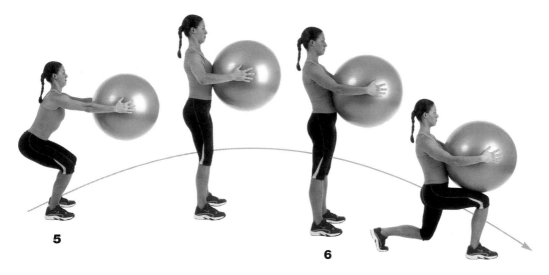

5

6

5 Progress to pressing the ball out as you squat and pulling the ball toward your chest as you stand up. Do 12 repetitions.

6 Holding the ball close to your chest, lunge your right foot forward so that your knee is over your ankle. Bend and lower your left knee toward the floor.

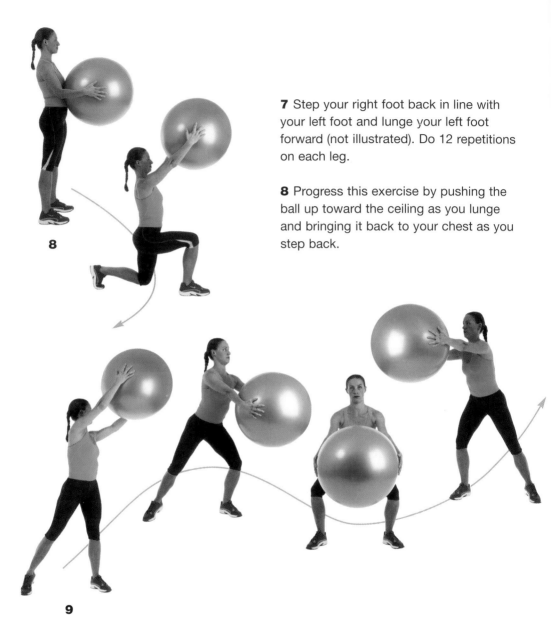

7 Step your right foot back in line with your left foot and lunge your left foot forward (not illustrated). Do 12 repetitions on each leg.

8 Progress this exercise by pushing the ball up toward the ceiling as you lunge and bringing it back to your chest as you step back.

9 Set your feet a little more than hip-width apart. Swing the ball from one side to the other and then swing it in a full circle in one direction and then the other. Do about 8 repetitions of both moves.

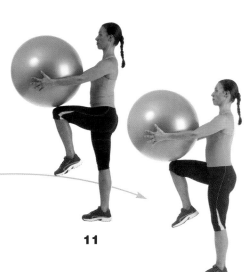

10

11

10 With the ball in your hands or on the floor, march on the spot for about a minute. You can move the ball toward and away from your chest as you march, or lift and lower it.

11 Holding the ball in front of you, lift alternate knees up to touch the ball for about a minute.

12

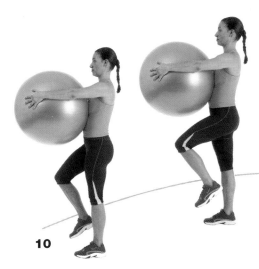

12 Progress this exercise by lifting alternate legs diagonally across your body as you swing the ball across to the hip of the raised leg.

13 Once you are warmer sit on the ball and do the pelvic tilts and single-leg balance exercises described in the Seated chapter, pages 49–51 (not illustrated).

standing

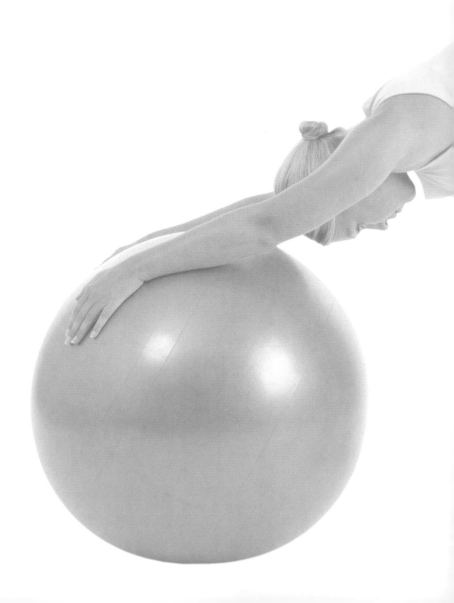

- rotator cuff
- shoulder stretch
- upper back stretch
- rotary torso stretch
- lateral torso stretch
- hip flexor stretch
- forward bending torso stretch
- hamstring stretch
- hip abductor stretch
- forward bending lat stretch

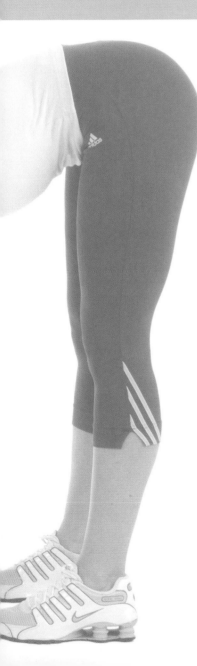

working with the ball in a standing position

Standing exercises are usually very functional because we live a lot of our lives and carry out many tasks standing up. The more we mimic daily movements, focusing on posture, alignment, and the recruitment of muscles when we work out and exercise, the better and more easily we carry out those tasks when we do them in daily life.

Postural alignment is a vital component in all the standing exercises as well as in the other exercise positions. All the start or set-up positions will have postural reminders but there are some basic cues that should be remembered for all positions.

Your feet should be hip-width apart and facing forward, with ankle, knee, hip, and shoulder joints level. Your knees and ankles should lie directly under your hips and your knees should be very slightly bent so they are never over-extended or "locked out."

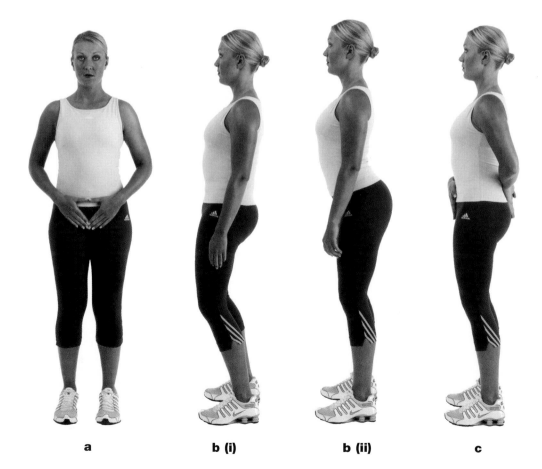

a   b (i)   b (ii)   c

It is important to check the position of your head, especially your chin, as this can affect the position of your neck. If you look at people in profile you will often see chins that jut out and protrude forward. This should be avoided as it pulls the head forward and the neck out of alignment. Instead, draw your chin toward the base of your skull, ensuring that it is parallel to the floor. This will lengthen your neck and keep your head in the correct position. Also check that your head is not tilting right or left but sitting centrally between your shoulders. The crown of your head should face the ceiling and your eyes should be looking straight ahead. Imagine a wire or thread emerging from the center of the crown of your head and attaching to the ceiling.

These cues may change slightly relative to changes in joint position as the exercises go from standing to seated to prone, and so on, but most will remain the same. Always focus on your posture and alignment before you start the exercise and then again as you are doing the exercise.

Don't forget to stabilize your core muscles as described earlier, and remember that the condition and stability of your torso affects what you can do and how you do it. The order should be a) activate transverse; b) engage your pelvic floor; c) movement.

a Your pelvis should be in "neutral." This means that your right and left hip bones, which you can feel if you press your fingers onto the front of your hip, and your pubic bone make up a triangle that should lie flat. If you imagine each point as a headlight, all three should shine onto the same surface.

b Neutral is somewhere between having your pelvis tilted too far back, as when you tuck your tailbone underneath you and flatten out your lower back (i), and tilted too far forward, as when you tuck your pubic bone backward and exaggerate the curve in your lower back (ii).

c If you place one hand on your pubic bone, fingers facing down, and one on your tailbone, both sets of fingers should point down toward the floor.

d If your pelvis is in neutral, your lower back should be as well. Your spine should have a natural "S" curve. Your chest should be "open," which comes from having your shoulders pressed down, away from your ears and your shoulderblades coming together slightly and easing down your back. Your shoulderblades should rest against your ribcage and your ribcage should close in as opposed to flaring out. We often forget that the neck is a part of the spine and should be long, with a natural slight concave curve.

d

squat against the wall

easy

benefits Doing your squats against a wall means you have to use the weight of your body to stabilize the ball against the wall as well as stabilize your body against the ball. It is a double challenge.

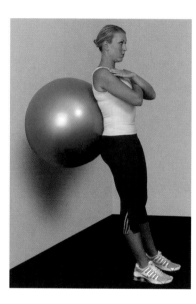
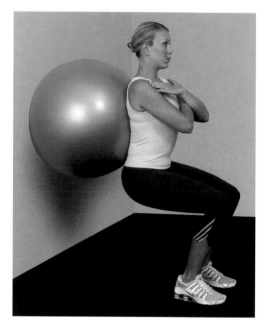

1 Place the ball against your lower back and rest it against the wall. Place your feet hip-width apart and walk your feet slightly forward so that you press more weight into the ball. Open your chest by pressing your shoulders down and squeezing your shoulderblades into the ball. Cross your arms over your chest so that your fingers rest on the opposite shoulders. Slowly bend your knees to a 90° angle, keeping your hips back. Your knees should stop directly over your ankles. Gently lift out of the squat, still keeping your hips back, and return to the start position.

2 Try 12 to 16 repetitions. Start by taking 4 counts to lower and another 4 to lift. Once your technique is excellent, try reducing the counts to 2 and 2.

tips

■ Make sure that that your knees are in line with your toes throughout the movement and that your chest remains open.

single leg squat against the wall

moderate

benefits Anything done on one leg introduces an element of balance that may not be there when a movement is done standing on both legs. This demands an additional layer of skill and strength when done properly. The amount of stabilization required also increases.

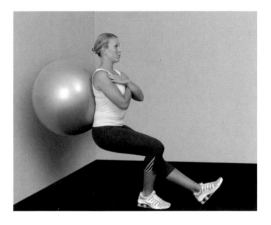

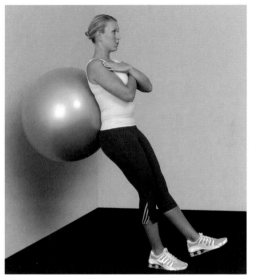

1 Position the ball as for the squat against the wall exercise and lift one foot off the floor. Hold the lifted foot clear of the floor as you move in and out of the squat.

tips

■ Try to ensure that the foot on the floor faces straight forward and does not start turning out or in.
■ Check that both hips are facing forward.

lunge against the wall

easy

benefits Lungeing is another good "compound" exercise that works different muscle groups of the legs simultaneously. It creates better synergy between these muscles that function together and depend on each other in daily life. It is always preferable that training or workout routines reflect real life muscle relationships.

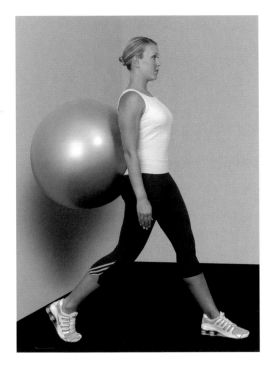

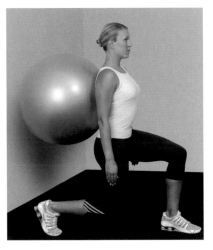

2 Push your body into the ball, bend both knees, and lower your body toward the floor, allowing the ball to roll up your back. Straighten your legs to return. Aim for 16 repetitions on each side, lowering and lifting in 4 counts. Then reduce to 2 counts on each phase.

1 Stand with one foot in front of the other. Lift the heel of your back foot so that you are standing on the ball of your foot. Place the ball behind your lower back and rest it against the wall. Keep your arms by your sides or let your hands rest on your front thighs.

tips

■ Check that your front knee stays in line with your front foot and that your knee is above your ankle when lungeing.
■ Keep your chest open and shoulders down throughout.

heel raise

easy

benefits This exercise strengthens and tones the calf muscles. Exercising calves can add shape and tone to a noticeable area of the legs.

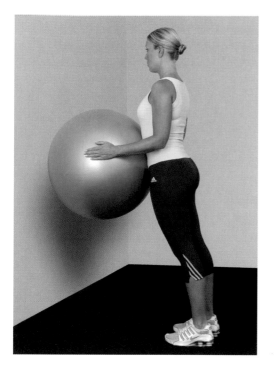
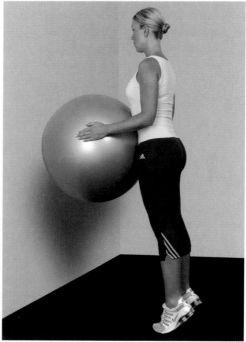

1 Place the ball against your torso and rest it against the wall. Check that your feet are parallel and both are facing straight toward the wall. Step your feet back so that they are behind your shoulders.

2 Gently lift and lower your heels with control, making sure that your heels touch the floor on every release. Start with 10 to 12 repetitions and work your way up to 16 repetitions.

tips

- Make sure that your feet remain parallel.
- Try to keep your weight over your big toes.
- Avoid rolling out over your ankles.

moving hip hinge

easy

benefits This exercise mimics the correct position for lifting a heavy object when it is not appropriate to bend your knees and kneel down to lift—for example, when taking something heavy out of the trunk of a car. This exercise helps strengthen the back while teaching good lifting technique.

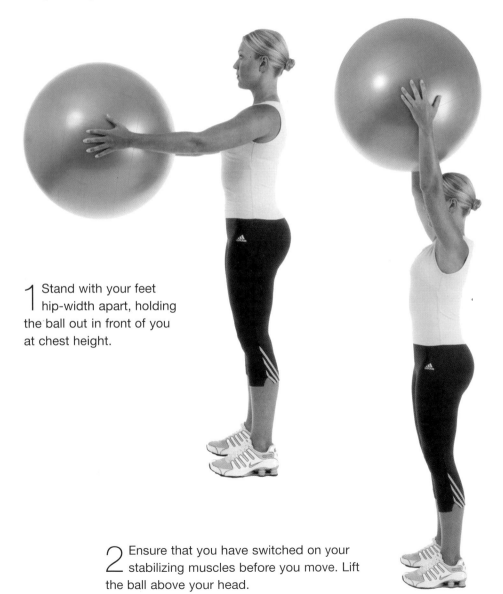

1 Stand with your feet hip-width apart, holding the ball out in front of you at chest height.

2 Ensure that you have switched on your stabilizing muscles before you move. Lift the ball above your head.

3 Keeping your spine long and your arms straight, bend from the hips to touch the ball to the floor. Ensure your body weight is taken evenly through your feet and that you do not rock back onto your heels.

tips

■ Try to maintain a natural curve in the lower back while pulling your navel toward your spine.

■ Think about keeping your shoulders down, away from your ears, even when you lift your arms.

■ You can bend your knees slightly as you bend over, if your hamstrings (back of thighs) are tight.

4 Without rounding your back, slowly unhinge from your hip joint to return to the start position. Repeat this 8 times in a slow, controlled manner.

lat stretch against the wall

easy

benefits This exercise will stretch and lengthen the lats. Tight lats can affect your posture and the quality of your movement.

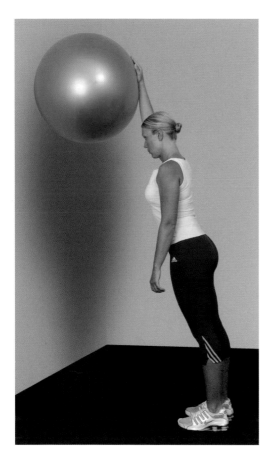

1 Stand facing the wall and place the ball against it at shoulder height. Support the ball on the wall with one hand and take a step back. Place your other hand by your side. Roll the ball up the wall. Lean your body toward the wall until you feel a stretch in the lats. Hold the position for 3 to 5 deep breaths.

tips

■ Move the ball around until you feel a good stretch below the shoulderblades.
■ Check that your shoulders and shoulderblades continue to draw away from your ears.

rotator cuff

easy

benefits The rotator cuff muscles in the shoulder are small muscles that allow the arms to rotate internally and externally. Weak rotators will have an effect on the function and strength of the shoulder joint as a whole.

1 Stand in a neutral position. Hold the ball overhead.

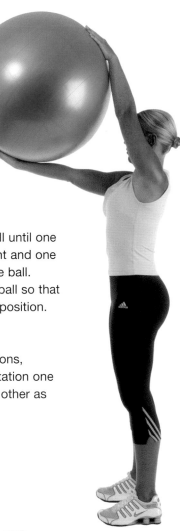

2 Rotate the ball until one hand is in front and one hand is behind the ball. Slowly rotate the ball so that the hands switch position.

3 Do 16 repetitions, counting a rotation one way and then the other as one repetition.

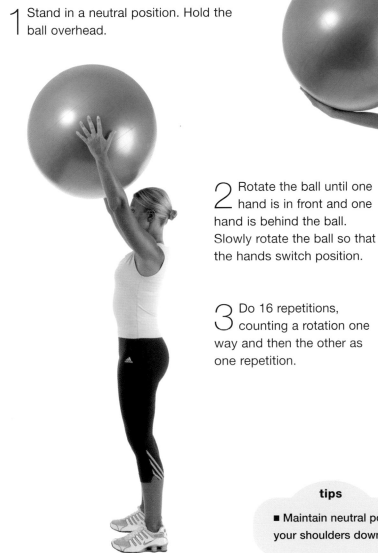

tips

■ Maintain neutral position and keep your shoulders down.

shoulder stretch

easy

benefits Whenever muscles are worked they should also be stretched out to maintain good muscle fiber length. Shortened fibers may, over time, affect posture and function.

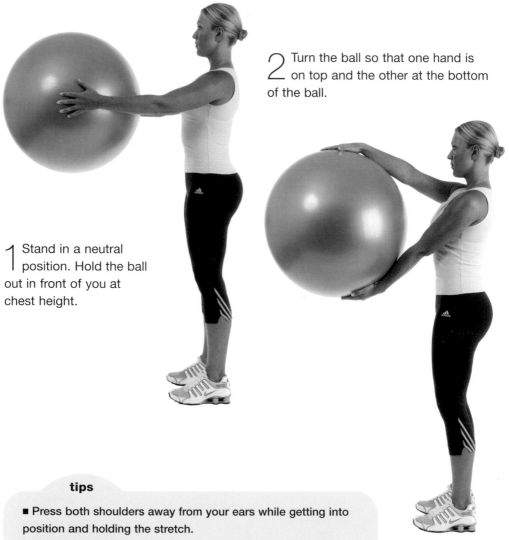

2 Turn the ball so that one hand is on top and the other at the bottom of the ball.

1 Stand in a neutral position. Hold the ball out in front of you at chest height.

tips

■ Press both shoulders away from your ears while getting into position and holding the stretch.

■ Keep both hips facing forward throughout the movement.

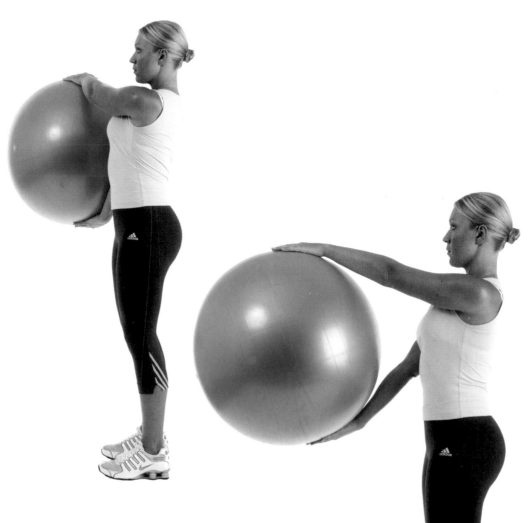

3 Slowly pull the ball across the body to stretch the back of the shoulder. Hold for 3 to 5 deep breaths.

4 Return to the start position and rotate the ball in the other direction to work the other side.

upper back stretch

easy

benefits This exercise relieves tension and tightness across the upper back.

1 Stand with your feet hip-width apart. Place the ball on your thighs and bend your knees.

2 Lengthen your arms over the front of the ball and round your upper back.

3 Separate your shoulderblades and draw your chest away from the ball. Hold for 3 to 5 deep breaths.

tip

■ Relax your chin onto your chest to involve the neck in the stretch.

rotary torso stretch

easy

benefits This exercise helps stretch the quadratus lumborum, the lats, trapezius, and obliques, and, of course, the muscles that allow the spine to rotate. This helps with mobility of the spine because the tighter muscles are, the more restricted movement will be.

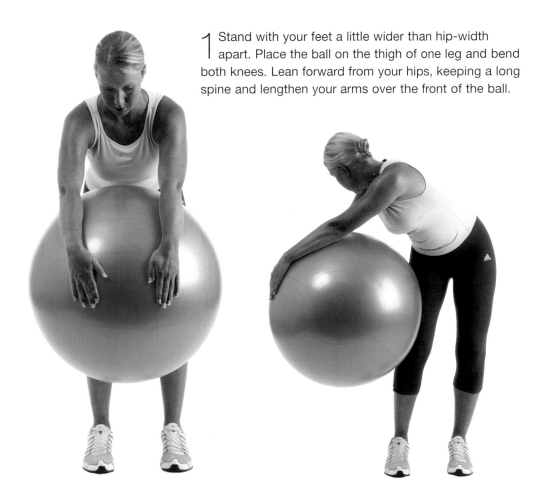

1 Stand with your feet a little wider than hip-width apart. Place the ball on the thigh of one leg and bend both knees. Lean forward from your hips, keeping a long spine and lengthen your arms over the front of the ball.

tip

■ Keep your feet and hips facing forward throughout the movement.

2 Roll the ball around to the side of your thigh as you turn toward the back, looking over your shoulder as far as you can. Turn back to face forward and then repeat on the other side. Hold for 3 to 5 deep breaths.

lateral torso stretch

easy

benefits This exercise lengthens the muscles that run down the side of the body and thereby allows the torso to feel longer.

1 Place your feet a little wider than hip-width apart. Place the ball against one side of your waist and hips.

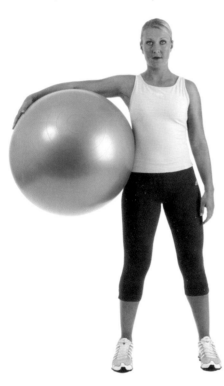

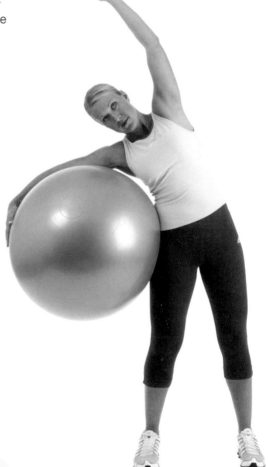

tips

■ Check that your hips are still over your knees and have not pressed out to one side.
■ Even though your arm is lifted, try to press your shoulders down away from your ears.

2 Drape your body sideways over the ball and extend your free arm overhead. Hold for at least 3 to 5 deep breaths.

hip flexor stretch

easy

benefits Tight hip flexors can cause the pelvis to tilt forward, throwing the pelvis and spine out of proper alignment. They get tight from all the work they do as we move—even simple walking—as well as from sitting for long periods.

1 Stand with the ball behind you and place one foot on top of the ball, front facing down.

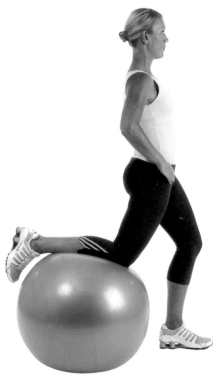

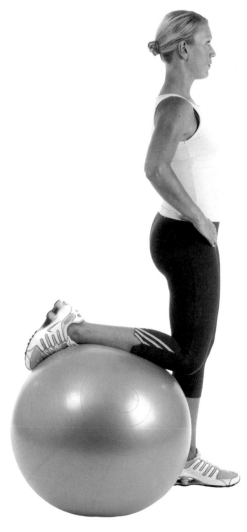

2 Maintain a neutral spine and roll the ball back until you feel a stretch in the front of the hip joint. Hold the position for 3 to 5 deep breaths.

tips

- Check that the knee of your standing leg is slightly bent.
- Keep your hips facing forward.
- Tuck your tailbone under slightly.

forward bending torso stretch

moderate

benefits Being a compound stretch, this exercise engages various muscles in the torso, including the rear shoulder and chest, simultaneously. The biceps may also get a stretch, depending on your flexibility.

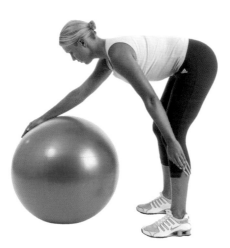

1 Place the ball on the floor in front of you. Take a wide stance and bend forward from your hips. Bend your knees and place one hand and forearm onto the ball.

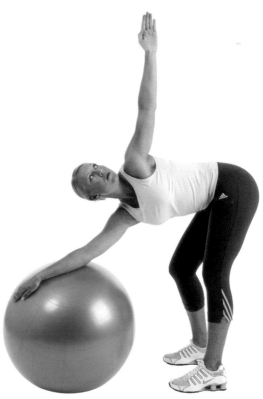

2 Gently roll the ball across your body as you rotate the spine and pull the other arm up behind you. Turn your head toward your raised arm. As the ball rolls across toward one leg, straighten this leg, keeping the other bent.

3 Roll the ball back in front of you, bending both legs again, and switch arms to stretch the other side. Hold for 3 to 5 deep breaths.

tips

- Ensure that the stretch happens through your torso rather than your hips or legs.
- You can support your body more by placing the second hand on your thigh, or bend your elbow and have that arm rest in the small of your back.

hamstring stretch

easy

benefits The hamstrings are another group of muscles that do lots of work and need a good stretch because of that. Sitting for long periods will also affect the length of these muscles. Tight hamstrings will tend to tilt the pelvis backward, out of the desired alignment, which will have an adverse affect on posture.

1 Stand with the ball in front of you and the heel of one foot on top of the ball.

tips

- Try to keep your standing leg and hips facing the ball.
- Your hips should always be level.
- Even if you have to start with a slight bend in your knee, the leg on the ball should eventually be straight.
- Check that your shoulders don't start to round as you lean forward.

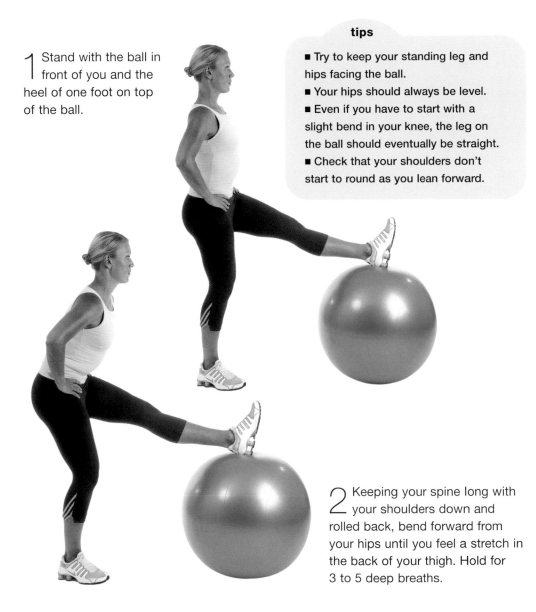

2 Keeping your spine long with your shoulders down and rolled back, bend forward from your hips until you feel a stretch in the back of your thigh. Hold for 3 to 5 deep breaths.

hip abductor stretch

moderate

benefits This exercise stretches the outer thigh muscles and will involve the external rotators to some extent.

1 Stand with the ball in front of you and place the heel of one foot on top of the ball.

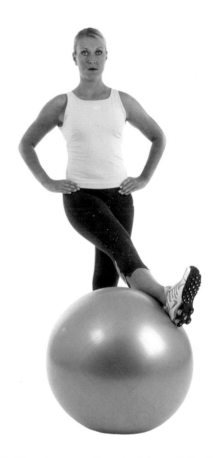

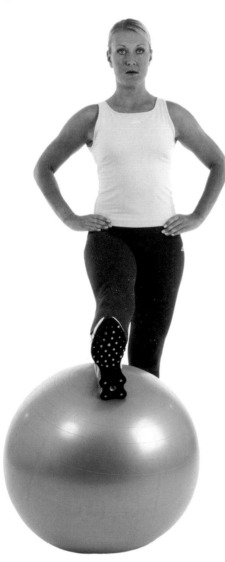

2 Keeping your leg straight, roll the ball to one side past the midline of your body. Hold for 3 to 5 deep breaths. Repeat on the other side.

tip

■ Keep your shoulders, chest and hips facing forward.

forward bending lat stretch

easy

benefits This exercise helps lengthen the lats. Tight lats affect posture, functioning of the back, and the range of movement of the arms.

1 Start in a wide stance. Bend your knees and fold over from your hips to place your hands on the ball in front of you.

2 Roll the ball away from you until you feel a pull through your lats. Straighten your legs if you can. Hold for 3 to 5 deep breaths.

tips

■ Make sure you do not lock out your knees when you straighten your legs.
■ Lengthen your spine from your tailbone to the base of your skull and try to keep it in neutral.

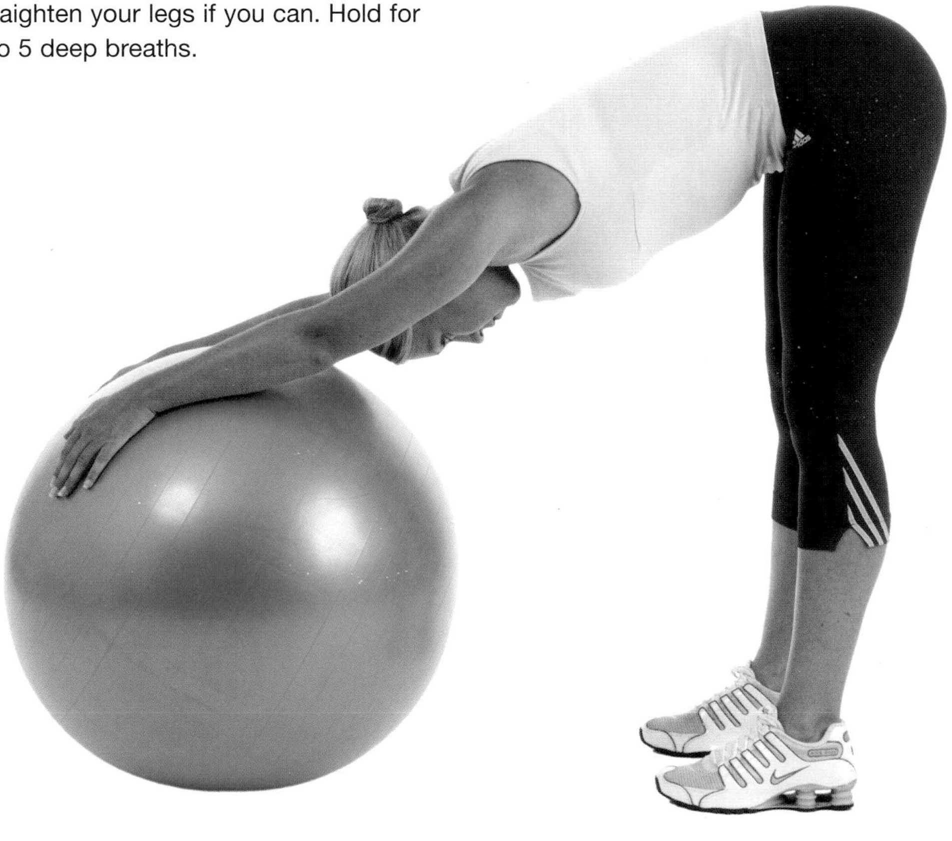

chapter 3

seated

- pelvic tilt
- lateral pelvic tilt
- single leg balance

- knee extension
- opposition arm to leg balance
- passive hamstring stretch
- active hamstring stretch
- adductor squeeze
- seated walk

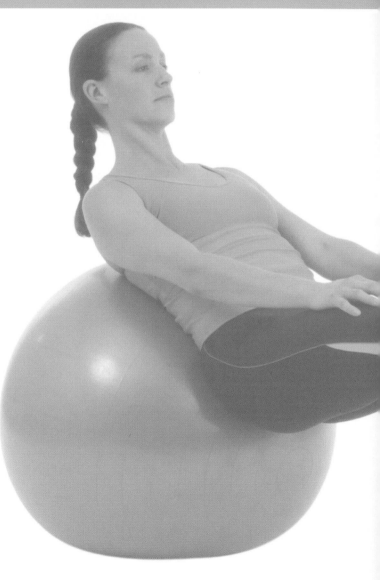

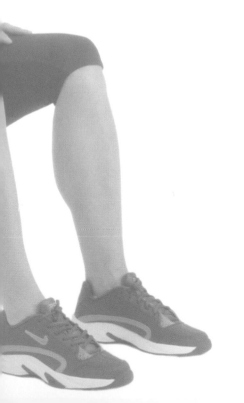

working with the ball in a seated position

Some of the postural points change with the change of position from standing to being seated. The key ones are that in a seated position the hip and knee joints are flexed or bent, usually to about 90°. When you sit on the ball your thighs should be parallel with the floor. Another good way to measure this is by checking that your knees are in line with or slightly above your hips. Always ensure that you have a ball that is the right height for you.

As you sit on the ball, the crown of your head should have an imaginary connection to the ceiling, almost like a magnet, or think of a strong thread or wire running up your spine, through your crown, and attaching you to the ceiling. Feel your spine lengthen as you think of the thread, still keeping the natural curves you should have in your spine, especially in your lower back. Shoulders are always down and slightly back to open your chest. Shoulderblades are set down against your ribcage. Your pelvis should be in neutral which, in a seated position, means the hip bone and pubic bone triangle is flat and facing forward. Knees and hips should be in line and knees should be directly over ankles. Your feet should be parallel and facing forward.

It is easy enough to move to sit on the ball but always check that it has not rolled away before you sit down. Use one hand to hold it while you sit down on it.

> The text will sometimes refer to your "sitting bones." These are the two bony points at the bottom of the pelvis. Sit on the floor or a chair and place your hands under your butt. Move your pelvis forward and backward. You should feel a bony protrusion beneath each buttock. These are the "sitting bones" or "ischial tuberosity."

The following exercises are all based on a strength or flexibility element. Often, though, any one exercise will require elements of both to be performed well.

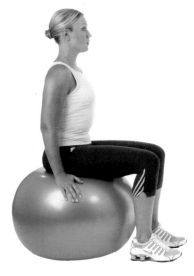

left> **Sitting correctly on the ball involves having a long, naturally curved, spine, thighs parallel with the floor, and the knees directly over the ankles and in line with the hips.**

pelvic tilt

easy

benefits This simple starting exercise is designed to get the mind switched on and connected to the body so that the body is aware of what it is doing and what is happening inside and out relative to posture and alignment in a seated position.

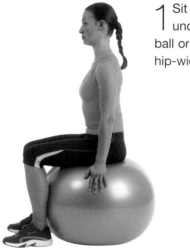

1 Sit on the center of the ball with your ankles under your knees, resting your hands on the ball or on the front of your thighs. Have your feet hip-width apart, shoulders down, and chest open.

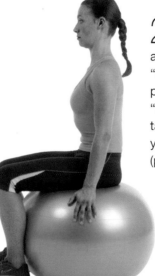

2 Lengthen your spine so that you are sitting on your "sitting bones" and your pelvis and spine are in "neutral." Tuck your tailbone under so that your pelvis moves back (posterior tilt).

3 Return to the start position then move your pelvis forward so that the arch in your back is exaggerated (anterior tilt). Return to neutral. Repeat 15 times in a slow, controlled manner.

tip

■ Avoid moving the legs. All the movement should happen through the pelvis and spine.

lateral pelvic tilt

easy

benefits This exercise promotes a heightened body awareness and improvement of posture and alignment.

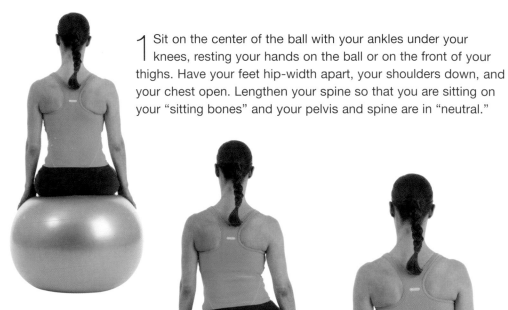

1 Sit on the center of the ball with your ankles under your knees, resting your hands on the ball or on the front of your thighs. Have your feet hip-width apart, your shoulders down, and your chest open. Lengthen your spine so that you are sitting on your "sitting bones" and your pelvis and spine are in "neutral."

2 Hitch your pelvis up to the right so that you are almost lifting your right "sitting bone" off the ball.

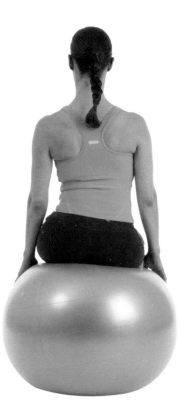

tips

■ Once you have practiced both pelvic tilts, you can put them together and draw a circle with your pelvis as a mobility exercise.

■ Always return to the neutral start position.

3 Return to neutral and do the same on the left side. Repeat 15 times in a slow, controlled manner.

single leg balance

easy/moderate

benefits This is a simple move that can actually be quite difficult if balance training has not been a part of a training regime. We often hear about the risk of elderly people falling, partly as a result of poor balance. Maintaining balance is a skill that we need increasingly as we get older, and we are more liable to lose it if we don't train it. For more of a challenge take your hands off the ball.

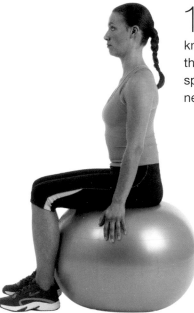

1 Sit on the center of the ball with your ankles under your knees, resting your hands on the sides of the ball. Your spine and pelvis should be in neutral position.

2 Lift one foot slightly off the floor and hold the position for 3 deep breaths.

tips

■ Your pelvis and spine should be in neutral throughout this exercise.
■ Try to minimize the movement of the ball as much as possible.

3 Repeat on the other side. Repeat the whole sequence again 5 times.

knee extension

easy/moderate

benefits This exercise strengthens the quads, which work to extend the knee and so are much in demand in walking and running activities, climbing stairs and hills, and so on. You can make the exercise more difficult by taking your hands off the ball.

1 Sit in neutral position as for the single leg balance and lift your foot off the floor. Contract your quads to straighten your leg.

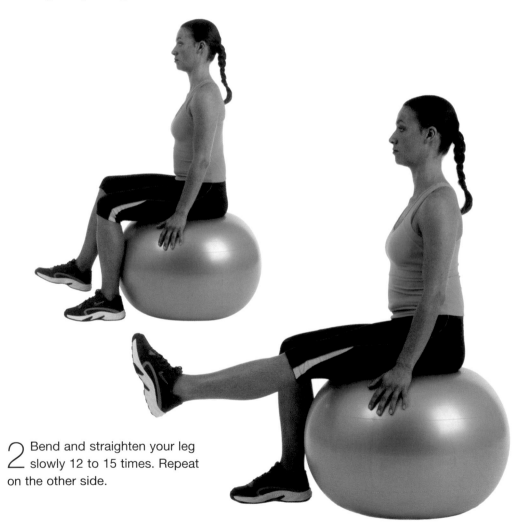

2 Bend and straighten your leg slowly 12 to 15 times. Repeat on the other side.

opposition arm to leg balance

moderate

benefits We walk, run, and play various sports using the upper and lower body (essentially the arms and legs) in opposition. This means that as your right leg moves forward as you walk, so does your left arm, and vice versa. It is the body's natural way of balancing and essential to good function. Training can improve the relationship between opposing sides and muscle groups so that they work more effectively and efficiently together.

1 Set up as if to perform the knee extension in the previous exercise

2 Extend the knee of one leg as you lift the opposing arm. Release the arm and leg while still holding neutral. Repeat on the other side.

3 Repeat the whole sequence 8 times, maintaining each lift for 2 breaths.

tip

■ If needed, use the nonlifting arm to hold onto the side of the ball.

passive hamstring stretch

easy

benefits The hamstrings are commonly some of the tightest muscles in the body and they easily become shortened, especially in people who sit a lot. Stretching helps lengthen them and reduces the risk of cramp through overactivity of the muscle fibers.

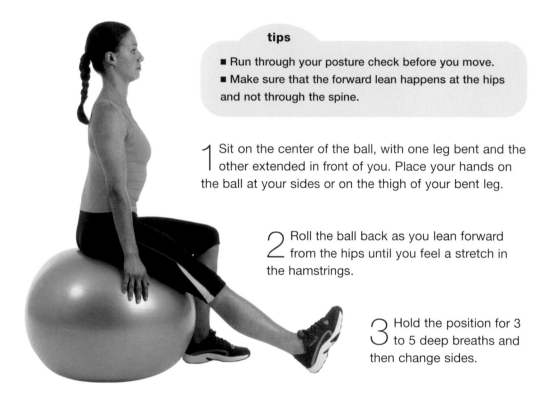

tips

- Run through your posture check before you move.
- Make sure that the forward lean happens at the hips and not through the spine.

1 Sit on the center of the ball, with one leg bent and the other extended in front of you. Place your hands on the ball at your sides or on the thigh of your bent leg.

2 Roll the ball back as you lean forward from the hips until you feel a stretch in the hamstrings.

3 Hold the position for 3 to 5 deep breaths and then change sides.

variations

- You can make the stretch a little more intense by extending both legs and stretching them at the same time.
- You can also involve the calf in this stretch by flexing your ankle(s) and pulling your toes toward you.

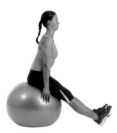

active hamstring stretch

moderate

benefits This exercise also lengthens the hamstrings but performing the stretch actively instead of passively involves the opposing muscle group too, which increases the overall workload of the exercise and enhances the synergy of the muscles.

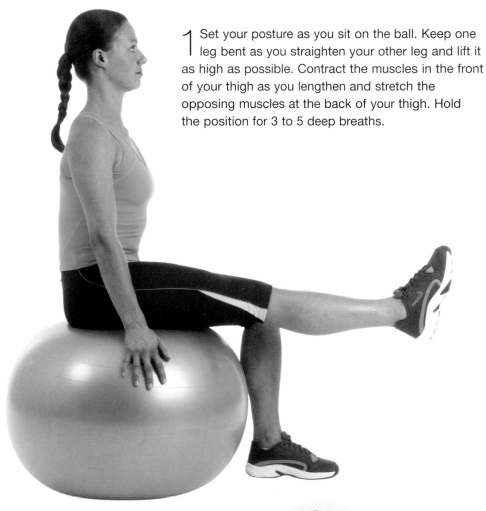

1 Set your posture as you sit on the ball. Keep one leg bent as you straighten your other leg and lift it as high as possible. Contract the muscles in the front of your thigh as you lengthen and stretch the opposing muscles at the back of your thigh. Hold the position for 3 to 5 deep breaths.

tips

■ Straighten the knee of your lifted leg as much as possible.
■ Maintain good postural alignment.

adductor squeeze

easy

benefits This exercise strengthens the inner thigh muscles within the range of movement allowed in the straddle position.

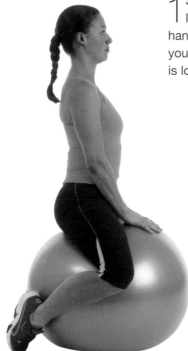

1 Sit on the center of the ball, straddling it with your legs and knees softly touching the sides and your hands lightly touching the front. Place your feet behind you with toes touching the floor. Ensure that your spine is long and your torso stabilized.

2 Slowly squeeze the ball as if you want to bring your inner thighs together. Hold the position for 5 to 8 seconds. Repeat 12 to 15 times.

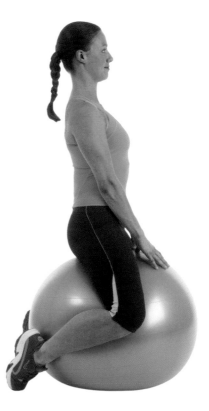

tip

■ Rather than holding the contraction, you can squeeze and release continuously for the same number of repetitions.

seated walk

moderate

benefits This exercise strengthens the legs and core muscles through working with the instability of the ball and movement of the body.

1 Sit on the front edge of the ball and walk your feet forward carefully, allowing your bottom and back to roll down the ball toward the floor.

tips

■ Your hands can rest on the front of your thighs or be at your sides.
■ Be aware of the feel of the ball on your back so that you don't walk too far.

2 As you walk back up, contract your abdominals, round your spine, and return to the start position.

half squat

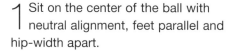

moderate

benefits As a "compound" exercise squats work most of the major leg muscles and some muscles of the hip joint. The hamstrings, quads and gluteus maximus are trained to build up moving strength while the inner and outer thigh muscles are trained to stabilize the legs and knee joint as the movement takes place. Other muscles stabilize the pelvis and the core. If done properly, it is one of the most efficient exercises, and so is very commonly used.

1 Sit on the center of the ball with neutral alignment, feet parallel and hip-width apart.

2 Rest your hands on the front of your thighs and lift your bottom about 2 inches (5cm) off the ball. Slowly sit back onto the ball. Repeat 12 to 15 times.

tips

■ Keep your knees and feet facing forward.

■ If the ball tends to roll away as you stand, use one hand to hold it in place. Switch hands halfway through.

back stretch

easy

benefits This exercise stretches the muscles along the whole length of the back. It also helps combat the constant compression effect of gravity.

tip

■ You should sense any tension easing out of your back and feel as though you can sit taller after the stretch.

1 Sit firmly on the center of the ball with your legs and feet hip-width apart and parallel. Link your hands together, palms facing toward you, in front of you at shoulder height, keeping your elbows slightly bent.

2 Push your arms away from you as you round your upper back. Ease your chin to your chest. Tuck your tailbone under to stretch your lower back as well. Hold the position for 3 to 5 deep breaths.

adductor stretch

easy

benefits This exercise lengthens and stretches the inner thigh muscles. This helps keep a balance between the strength and the flexibility of a muscle or muscle group.

tips

■ The knee on the bent leg should line up over your ankle.

■ Maintain a long spine.

1 Sit on the front edge of the ball, bending one leg to one side.

2 Straighten your other leg out to the other side. You should feel a stretch in the inner thigh of the straight leg. Hold the position for 3 to 5 deep breaths. Repeat on the other side.

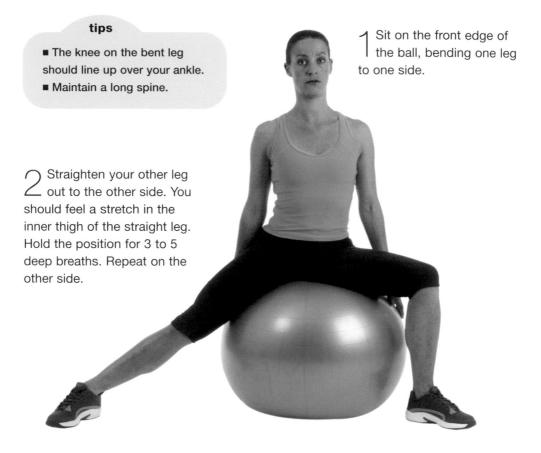

variation

■ Sit upright on the front edge of the ball and place your legs and feet out to either side. Place your hands on the inside of your upper thighs and press your knees out until you feel a stretch in your inner thighs. Hold the position for 3 to 5 deep breaths.

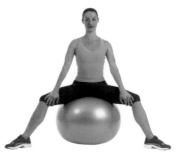

adductor triangle stretch

moderate

benefits This stretch is an inner thigh stretch but it involves the upper body and so helps with how the upper and lower body function together in terms of flexibility. The flexibility of the upper body, especially the shoulders and upper back, will affect the hips because some of the muscles of the back connect into the hip region.

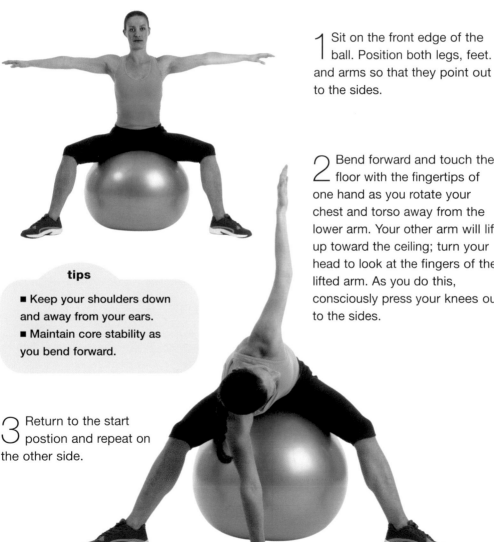

1 Sit on the front edge of the ball. Position both legs, feet. and arms so that they point out to the sides.

2 Bend forward and touch the floor with the fingertips of one hand as you rotate your chest and torso away from the lower arm. Your other arm will lift up toward the ceiling; turn your head to look at the fingers of the lifted arm. As you do this, consciously press your knees out to the sides.

tips

- Keep your shoulders down and away from your ears.
- Maintain core stability as you bend forward.

3 Return to the start postion and repeat on the other side.

hip flexor stretch

easy

benefits The hip flexors, which cross the front of the hip joint, are another group of muscles that become tight from sitting as well as from all movements that involve an element of hip flexion. They need to be stretched regularly to counterbalance the effects of everyday use.

1 Sit sideways on the edge of the ball with your front leg bent and your back leg straight out behind. Place your outside hand on your hip or your front thigh and your inner hand on the ball.

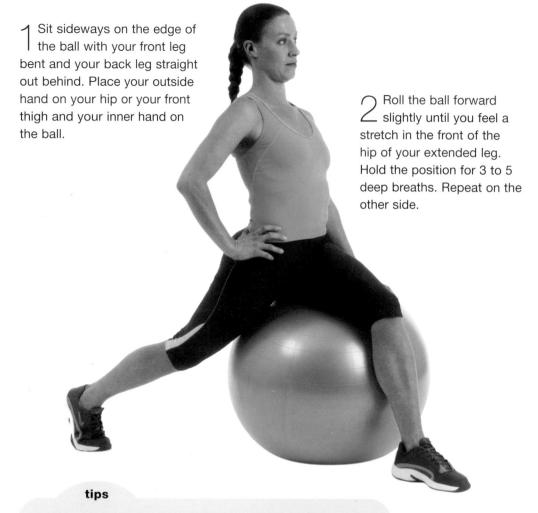

2 Roll the ball forward slightly until you feel a stretch in the front of the hip of your extended leg. Hold the position for 3 to 5 deep breaths. Repeat on the other side.

tips

- Tuck your hip under slightly rather than just leaning forward.
- The knee of your bent leg should be above your ankle.
- Both your knee and foot should be facing forward.

hip flexor with tibialis

moderate

benefits The muscles of the shin are rarely stretched but they are much used in walking as the heel is planted on the ground with the toes lifted. Stretching helps create more of a balance between the work, which contracts and shortens the muscle, and the stretch, which relaxes and lengthens the muscle.

1 Sit sideways on the edge of the ball with your front leg bent, your back leg straight out behind, and your back foot placed so that the front faces down toward the floor. Rest on the toenail of your big toe rather than on the flesh. Place your outside hand on your hip.

2 Roll the ball forward slightly until you feel a stretch in the front of the hip and the front of your ankle on the extended leg. Hold the position for 3 to 5 deep breaths. Repeat on the other side.

tip

■ Hold onto the ball with your inside hand for balance if necessary.

lateral torso stretch

easy

benefits This exercise stretches the sides of the body by lengthening the torso out of the hips, which helps with posture and body length.

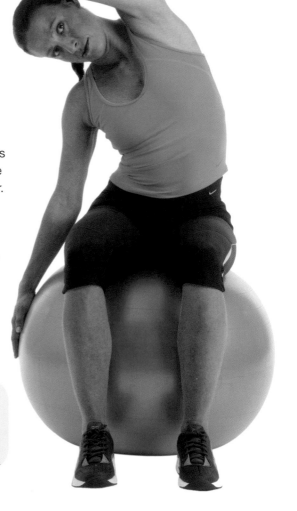

1 Sit on the center of the ball with your legs and feet hip-width apart and parallel. Steady yourself by placing one hand on the side of the ball.

2 Lengthen your other arm above your head and reach over to the other side. You can increase the intensity of this stretch by shifting your weight to the side as you let your hips drop toward the floor.

3 Return to the start position and do the same on the other side. Hold the position for 3 to 5 deep breaths.

tips

■ Avoid collapsing into the side that is bending.
■ Try to keep some distance between your hips and your ribs.

rotary stretch

easy

benefits Stretching should be done in all the planes of movement that muscles work in to maintain a balance between strength and stretch.

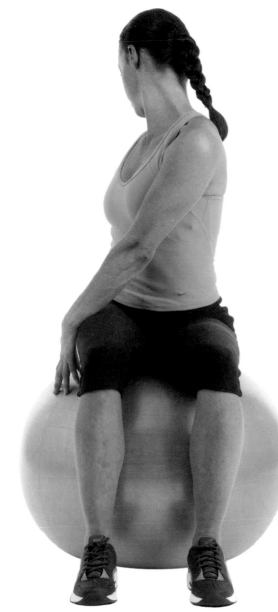

1 Sit on the center of the ball with your feet and legs hip-width apart. Ensure that you are sitting tall and that your pelvis is in a neutral position.

2 Place both hands on one side of the ball and rotate around as far as possible toward your hands so that you are looking over your shoulder. Hold the position for 3 to 5 deep breaths.

3 Return to neutral and repeat on the other side.

tip

■ Maintain an erect spine and neutral pelvis as you move and hold the stretch.

single arm chest stretch

easy

benefits If the chest is tight, the shoulders and upper back tend to be rounded and the arms turn into the body. This affects posture and if not addressed, can over years cause kyphosis, where a hump begins to form in the upper back.

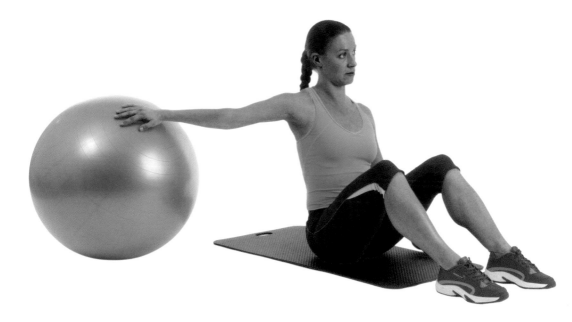

1 Sit on the floor with the ball beside you. Bend your knees and establish and maintain an upright posture.

2 Place one hand on the ball and roll it back until you feel a stretch in the chest and the front of the shoulder.

3 Hold the position for 3 to 5 deep breaths. Repeat on the other side.

tips

■ Keep your torso and head facing forward throughout.
■ Ensure that your spine remains lengthened.

glute stretch

easy

benefits This exercise stretches one of the main postural muscles. The glutes work very hard in all standing and moving activities.

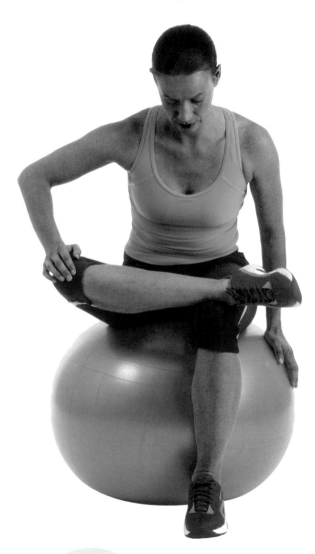

1 Sit on the center of the ball. Bend one knee and place the ankle of that leg on the thigh of the other leg. If your right leg is bent, place your right hand on your right thigh and your left hand on the ball. Keep your spine in neutral as you lean forward from your hip joint until you feel a stretch in the hip. Repeat on the other side.

tip

■ Place your hands lightly on the side of the ball for balance.

variation

■ Extend your arms out in front as an additional balance challenge.

triceps dip

easy

benefits The biceps and triceps are opposing muscle groups. The biceps are usually a lot stronger than the triceps because they are used more in daily activity. This sort of exercise can help redress the imbalance and thereby reduce any risk of injury.

1 Sit on the front edge of the ball. Place your hands on the ball behind you, fingers pointing toward your bottom.

tips

■ Try to make sure the movement is initiated through the arms and not through the hips.
■ When you have mastered the technique, speed up the timing of the exercise so that you take 2 counts to bend and 2 to straighten.

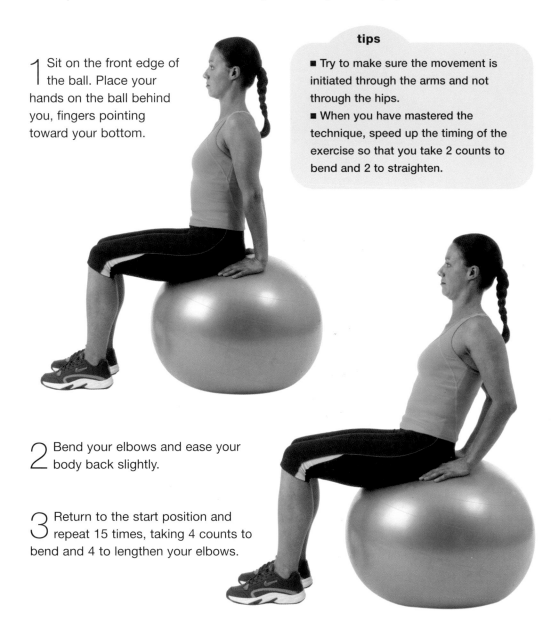

2 Bend your elbows and ease your body back slightly.

3 Return to the start position and repeat 15 times, taking 4 counts to bend and 4 to lengthen your elbows.

triceps dip

moderate

benefits The triceps are the muscles used when you place your hands on the arm of a chair to push yourself out of it. Many older people lose the ability to lift their body weight in this way and it affects their mobility and independence. Triceps should be trained to at least maintain the strength required to lift one's body weight.

1 Sit on the front edge of the ball. Place your hands on the ball behind you. Ease your bottom off the ball and hold it suspended in mid-air.

tips

■ Keep your hips near the ball so that your back almost brushes it as you lower your hips.

■ Speed up so that you take 2 counts to bend and 2 to straighten when you can do it faster and still maintain good technique at the same time.

2 Bend your elbows and lower your hips toward the floor. Slowly lift back up to the suspended position. Repeat 15 times taking 4 counts to bend and 4 to lengthen your elbows.

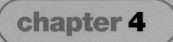

chapter 4

supine on
the ball

- incline abdominal curl
- abdominal curl
- oblique curl
- bridge
- bridge single leg balance

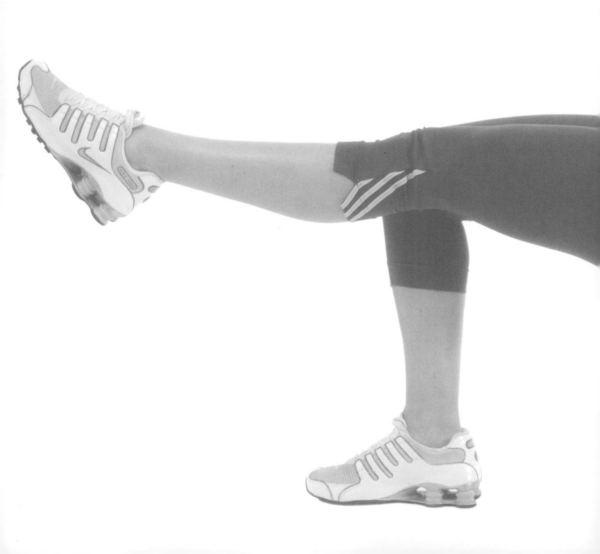

- chest stretch
- abdominal stretch
- pullover
- chest flye with dumbbells
- chest press with dumbbells
- lateral roll
- scapula retraction
- heel raise

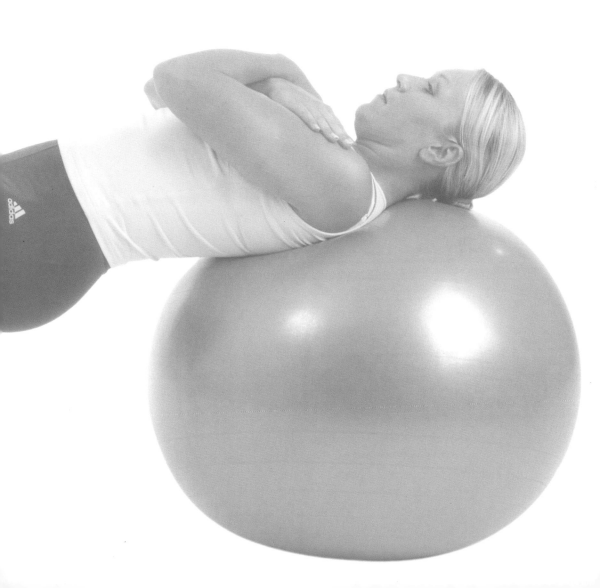

working on the ball in a supine position

The postural cues remain the same as already established in the Standing chapter, save that the knees and hip joint have changed position. "Supine" means "face up," so generally your face will be up toward the ceiling unless you are in an inclined position that sets you on more of a diagonal angle on the ball.

In any event, incline or straight supine, your knees will be bent and should still be directly over your ankles. Your knees should remain in line with your hips and your hips should be flat and open unless the exercise requires the hips to bend.

In order to move safely into a supine position, start by sitting on the ball (a). Walk your feet forward, away from the ball. Use your hands to steady the ball for as long as you can if you need additional support (b). Your body will travel down the ball as the ball rolls up your back (c). Stop when the ball is in the required position and set your starting posture (d).

To return to a seated position, walk your feet in toward the ball. As your body moves up the ball, the ball will roll down your back and under your hips. When walking the feet in, you will get to a stage when you can place your hands on the ball and use them to steady it as you roll up.

If you are exercising with bare feet, make sure that the surface you are on is not going to cause your feet to slip.

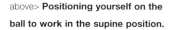

above> **Positioning yourself on the ball to work in the supine position.**

incline abdominal curl

easy

benefits This incline position requires more stabilization to take place through the legs as the exercise is done, but the intensity of the curl is less than if you were lying flat on the ball. You will be working your abdominals and legs at the same time.

1 Walk yourself into a seated position with the ball somewhat behind you rather than directly underneath you. Your hips will be slightly flexed. Check that your knees and ankles are hip-width apart and facing forward.

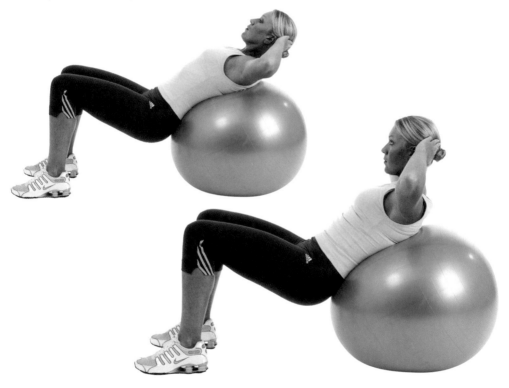

tips

■ The ball should not move.
■ Set your pelvis, shoulderblades and head/neck position before you move.
■ Placing your feet wider apart will make the movement easier.

2 Choose an appropriate arm position, depending on your strength level. Contract your abdominals to curl forward and lift your shoulderblades away from the ball. Slowly return to the start position. Repeat up to 10 times, taking 2 to 3 seconds to lift and lower your body.

abdominal curl

easy/moderate

benefits This exercise strengthens the abdominal muscles, particularly the rectus abdominus, which causes the spine to flex. If you also engage the deeper abdominals—the transverse abdominus—and the obliques, this will make the exercise even more effective. You will also find that your movement is more efficient and you don't have to do many curls to achieve a good abdominal workout.

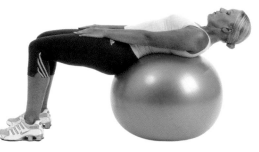

1 Set yourself in a lying position with your legs and feet hip-width apart. Have the ball positioned under your mid and upper back so that your body is in a fairly straight line out from the ball. Rest your hands on the front of your thighs.

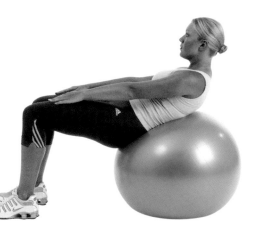

2 Curl yourself up by contracting your abdominals and sliding your hands down your thighs as your back lifts off the ball.

3 Slowly lower yourself back down and repeat up to 10 times, taking 2 to 3 seconds to lift and the same length of time to lower.

tips

■ Remember to pull up and engage your pelvic floor muscles, deep abdominals and back muscles for the best and most effective results.
■ Check that your head stays aligned and that you don't drop your chin toward your chest as you curl.

variations

■ You can progress this exercise by varying your arm position. Each progression adds a little more body weight to the movement. First try crossing your arms over your chest (a).

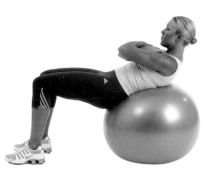

a

■ Next place your fingers lightly on your temples, with your elbows pointing out to the sides (b).

b

■ Finally, have both arms extended above your head (c) or extend one arm only and place your other hand behind your head to support it (not illustrated).

c

■ You can also use the legs to increase the body weight you have to work with. Any of the arm positions described can be done with one leg extended (d).

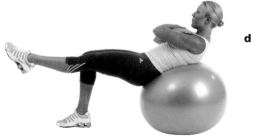

d

oblique curl

moderate

benefits This exercise works and strengthens the muscles that allow your torso to twist. Training these muscles can lower the risk of injury, such as pulling a back muscle during twisting movements.

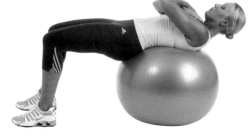

1 Lie flat on top of the ball or on a slight incline. Place your feet hip-width apart. Place your arms across your chest.

2 Gently lift your right shoulder across toward your left hip then release back to the start position. Take 4 seconds on each phase of the movement.

3 You should do up to 15 repetitions on each side.

variation

- Perform the exercise with your hands behind your head.

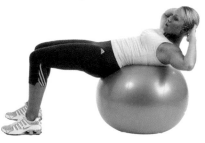

tips

- Focus on lifting your shoulder across so that it is not just your elbow that moves.
- You can do all the repetitions to one side and then change or you can alternate sides. Alternating gives one side a chance to rest.

bridge

easy

benefits A bridge done this way is a great exercise for training core stability. It strengthens core and postural muscles which in turn translates into better daily functioning and less risk of aches, pains, and injury.

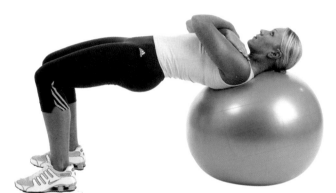

1 From a seated position take yourself into a bridge by walking your feet away from the ball. The lower you go, the farther the ball will roll up your back. You should stop when your knees are over your ankles and your body is in a straight line.

2 Keeping your spine long and head aligned, slightly bend at your hips and lower your bottom toward the floor.

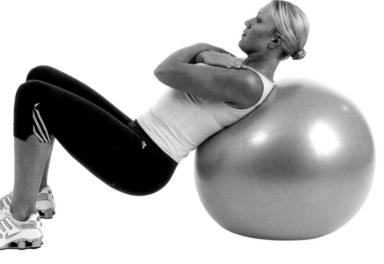

tips

■ Think about drawing your shoulderblades down your back and keeping them there as you move.
■ Your hips should remain parallel and not rock to either side.

3 Lift your hips up until they are back in line with your shoulders and knees. Repeat 15 times, taking 4 counts to lower and another 4 to lift.

bridge single leg balance

easy/moderate

benefits Balance is always an additional challenge for the body, especially in positions where balance is not usually required. Training for "balance" makes the body stronger from inside as it adapts to changes in stability. This exercise demands the ability to stabilize from most of the body's muscle groups, at the same time.

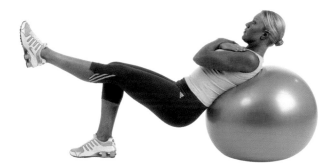

1 Lie on the ball with your knees directly over your ankles. Have your hips extended so that there is a straight line from your knee, through your hips, to your shoulders. Cross your arms over your chest, and lift the left foot.

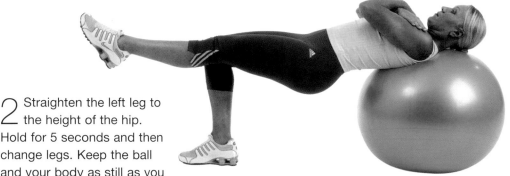

2 Straighten the left leg to the height of the hip. Hold for 5 seconds and then change legs. Keep the ball and your body as still as you can throughout.

variations

■ Once you can hold yourself still, lift the arm opposite to your lifted leg over your head, then hold the position for 5 seconds.

■ You can also start by extending your arm, then raising the leg.

tip

■ Try to ensure that your hips remain parallel and do not tilt your body to the right or left.

chest stretch

easy

benefits A tight chest can have an adverse effect on the ability to maintain good posture and alignment. The chest is one of the main areas of the body that can become tight in people who sit for many hours each day and work constantly on computers.

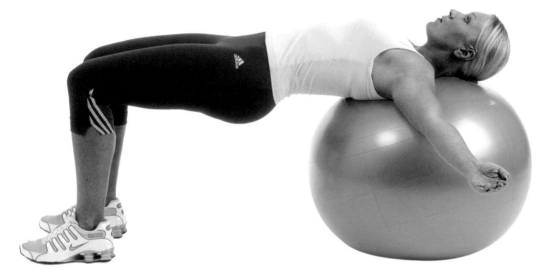

1 Take yourself into a lying position with the ball under your upper back and neck. Rest your head on the ball. Have your knees bent and feet firmly planted on the floor. Straighten out your hip joint.

2 Allow your arms to drop out to the sides, away from your body. You should feel a stretch in the chest and the front of your shoulders. Hold the position for at least 3 to 5 deep breaths.

tips

■ Press your back into the ball to assist your balance.
■ Try to hold the ball still.

abdominal stretch

easy

benefits All muscles can do with being lengthened from time to time. Tight or shortened superficial abdominals will affect posture because they cause the body to curl over. A stretch like this one will help address any tendency to rounded posture.

1 Have the ball rest under your lower back and hips as you walk from seated to lying.

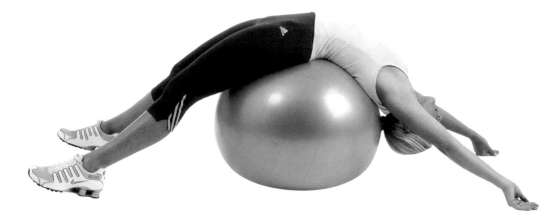

tip

■ Play with the positioning of the ball to get the best stretch possible.

2 Place your legs and feet hip-width apart and allow your body to drape over the ball. Your head should be hanging so that you can look at the wall behind you. You should feel the stretch along your stomach and the front of your hips. You can increase the stretch by taking your arms overhead.

pullover

moderate

benefits This exercise is done with dumbbells because the additional weight challenges the stabilizing strength of the body. The objective is to be able to take the arms and weight overhead without this causing the back to arch. It also addresses dynamic flexibility and mobility of the shoulder joint.

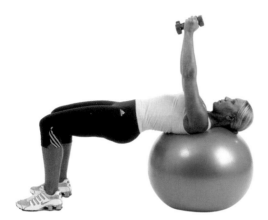

1 Take your weights in your hands and position yourself with the ball under your upper back so that your head can rest on it. Make sure that your legs and feet are aligned, hip-width apart. Start with your arms pointing up to the ceiling keeping a slight bend in your elbows.

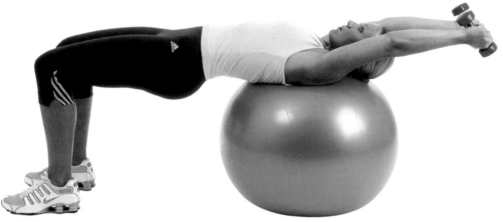

tips

- Work toward getting the inside of your upper arm beside your ears.
- Practice without any weight until you have the technique right.
- Use more weight as you get stronger.

2 Slowly lower your arms over your head until your inner arm is by your ears. Bring your arms back to start and repeat 15 to 20 times. Take 4 counts to complete each phase of the movement, checking that your spine stays in neutral position and your back does not arch.

chest flye with dumbbells

easy

benefits This exercise will work the chest muscles. The external resistance provided by the dumbbells should cause greater muscle fiber recruitment and thereby make the movement more intense than if done without dumbbells.

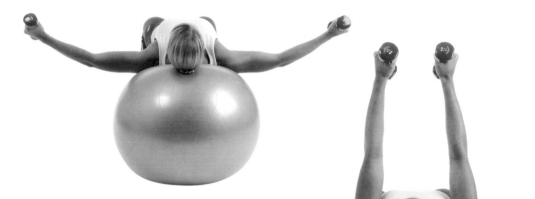

1 Take your weights in your hands and rest them on your chest or on your hips as you move from a seated to a lying position. Lie with the ball under your upper back, neck, and head and set your body in neutral. Position your arms straight out to the sides, palms facing up and your elbows very slightly bent.

tips

- Feel as though there is tone in your abdominals and back muscles all the time so that your body does not sag in the middle and the ball does not move.
- Start with light weights—maybe only 4½ lb (2 kg)—and progress to heavier weights as you grow stronger.
- You can progress the exercise by taking 2 counts instead of 4 to execute each phase of the movement.

2 Take 4 counts to bring the weights up so that your hands meet above your chest. Check that your wrists are straight.

3 Lower your arms back to the start position in 4 counts. Repeat at least 15 times.

chest press with dumbbells

easy

benefits This exercise strengthens the chest muscles.

1 Take your weights with you as you move from a seated position to set yourself lying on the ball. Place the ball under your upper back so that your head can also rest on it. Bend your elbows out to the sides so that they lie almost in line with your shoulders. Your palms are facing your feet and your wrists should be straight.

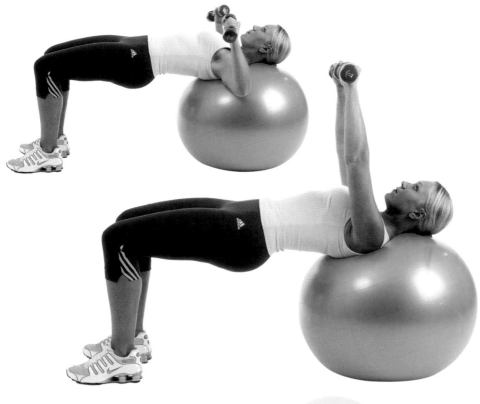

2 Take 4 counts to straighten your arms and lift the weights toward the ceiling. Lower your arms back to the bent position at the same pace. Do 15 to 20 repetitions.

tip

■ Even though your focus is on your arms, remember to think about holding the rest of your body in good alignment.

lateral roll

moderate

benefits This exercise challenges core stability in a supine position. As we move and function in different positions we should train the body to be strong in all those positions.

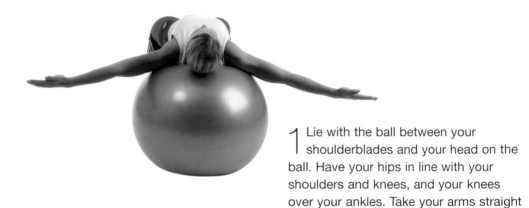

1 Lie with the ball between your shoulderblades and your head on the ball. Have your hips in line with your shoulders and knees, and your knees over your ankles. Take your arms straight out to the sides, palms facing up.

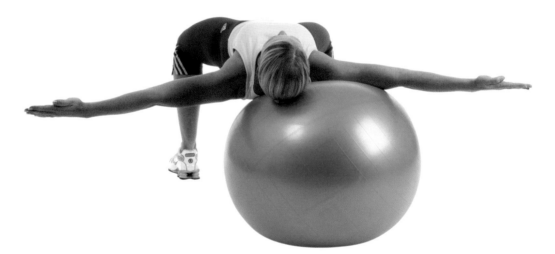

2 Slowly roll the ball sideways, allowing your feet to move with your body. Keep your hips in line with your shoulders and knees. Go as far as you can with good alignment and then roll to the other side.

tip

■ Keep your neck aligned with the rest of your body.

scapula retraction

moderate

benefits The rounded shoulder syndrome usually means that the muscles of the mid back are weak and don't hold the shoulderblades against the ribs or help draw the shoulders back. This exercise strengthens these muscles and thereby assists in improving posture.

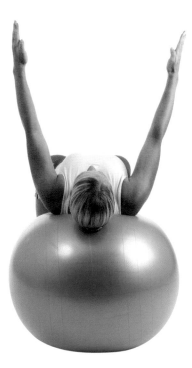

1 Place the ball under your upper back so that your head can rest on it. Keep your neck aligned with the rest of your spine, your hips, and your knees. Your knees should be directly over your ankles. Draw your shoulders away from your ears and raise your arms.

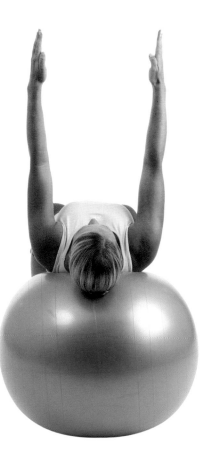

2 Lift your arms toward the ceiling. Press your shoulders down into the ball and squeeze your shoulderblades together slightly. Release and repeat 15 times.

tip

■ Feel as though you are opening your chest as you press your shoulders into the ball.

heel raise

easy/moderate

benefits Calf muscles should be strengthened and toned like all other muscles.

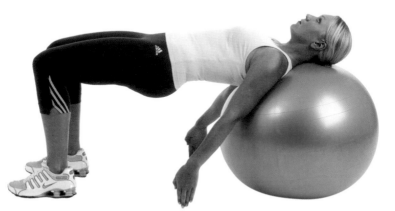

1 Walk yourself into a lying position until your head is resting on the ball. Have the rest of your body aligned and your fingers touching the floor for support.

variations

■ You can progress this exercise by lifting both heels together.
■ You can also try this exercise with your arms crossed over your chest

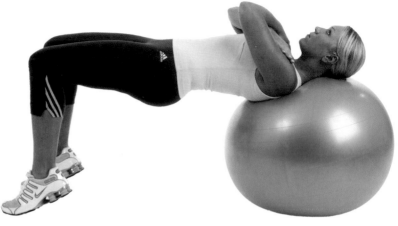

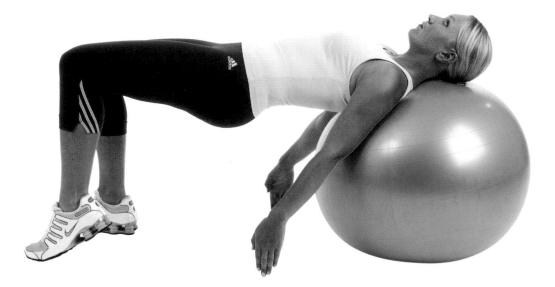

2 Keeping your toes on the floor, take 2 counts to lift one heel. Replace it and then lift the other.

3 Repeat at least 15 times on each leg. If you wish you can do all the repetitions on one side before you change to the other side.

tips

■ Keep your hips in line and ensure that they do not tilt, rock, or dip.

■ Make sure that you touch down with your heels after you have completed every lift.

supine on the floor

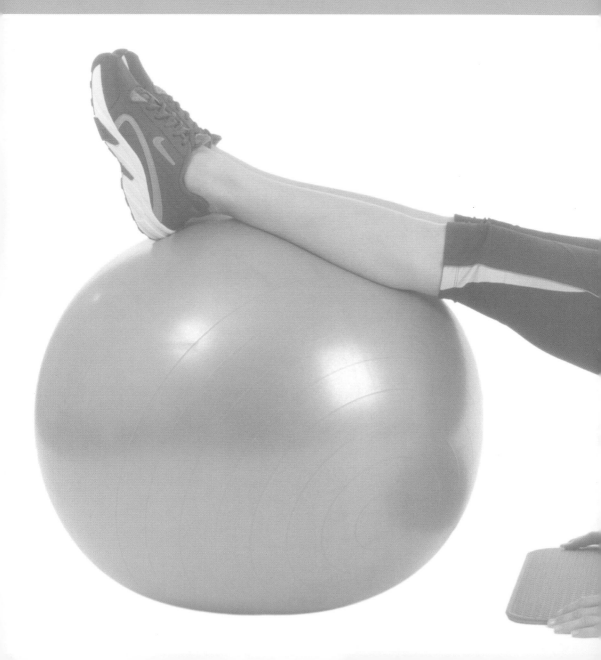

hip extension
leg curl
bridge leg curl
glute stretch
knee extension
shoulder rotator

● butterfly stretch
● rotary torso stretch
● active calf/hamstring stretch
● reverse curl
● leg press

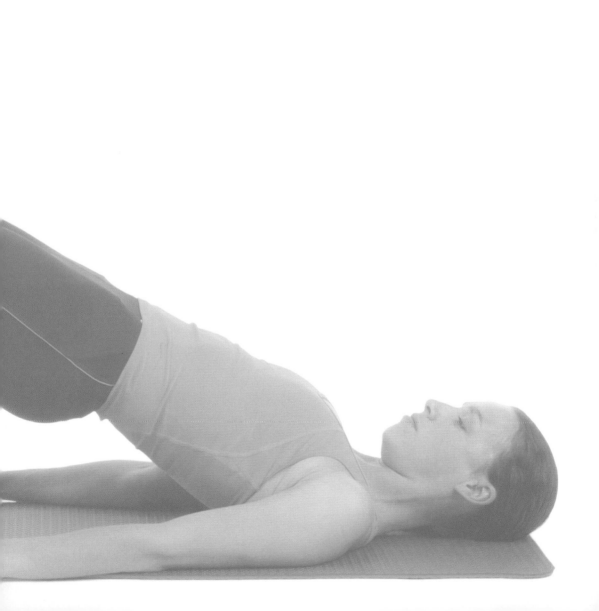

working on the floor in a supine position

You may need a mat or towel to work in this position, which requires you to lie on the floor on your back.

Most of the exercises described in this chapter require one or both legs to be bent, either resting on the ball or holding the ball. This affects the position of the lower back.

When the spine is in neutral, as it should be if you have both legs extended along the floor, you should have a natural concave curve in your lumbar spine (lower back).

When you bend your knees and lift your feet off the floor, as with these exercises, you should lightly press your lower back into the floor to reduce the stress and pressure that the lower back will be under when the legs are lifted. You must also set the core muscles to hold the position of the torso as the limbs move and to assist in keeping the body still where the exercise requires the body to be held in a certain position.

Apart from this change in positioning of the spine and legs, the postural cues outlined in the Standing chapter apply to working with the ball when lying supine on the floor.

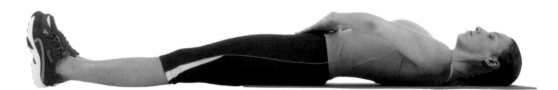

above> **The spine should be in neutral when you are supine on the floor.**

below> **You should lightly press the lower back into the floor when you raise your legs.**

hip extension

easy

benefits The hip flexors can get very tight, especially from desk jobs when one can be seated for many hours of the day with the hips bent. Hip extension exercises counteract the flexed position and bring some balance back into the hip flexor muscles.

1 Lie on the floor with your lower legs and feet on top of the ball. Keep your legs and feet aligned with your hips. Check that your knees and toes face up to the ceiling rather than turning out to the sides. Have your arms just out to the side of your body with your palms on the floor.

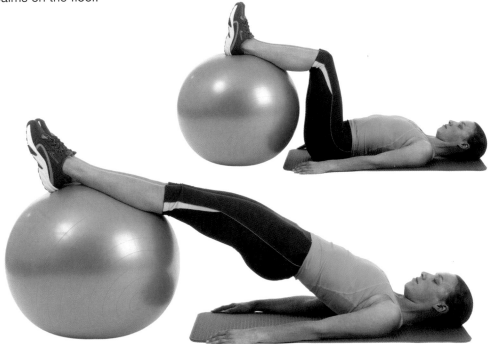

2 Contract your bottom to lift your hips so that your body weight is through the ball and across the top of your shoulders. There should be a straight line from your knee, through your hips, to your shoulders. Hold for 5 seconds and then release. Repeat at least 10 times.

tips

■ To avoid your hips turning out, put a small ball between your knees.
■ Relax your feet so that you are not overusing your calves in this exercise.

leg curl

easy

benefits This exercise works to strengthen the hamstrings and calves and improves the synergy of these muscle groups working together.

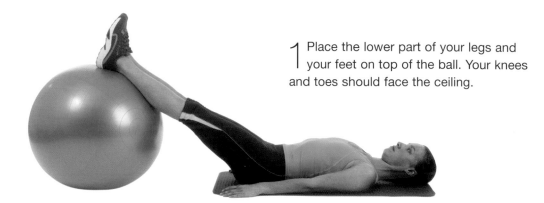

1 Place the lower part of your legs and your feet on top of the ball. Your knees and toes should face the ceiling.

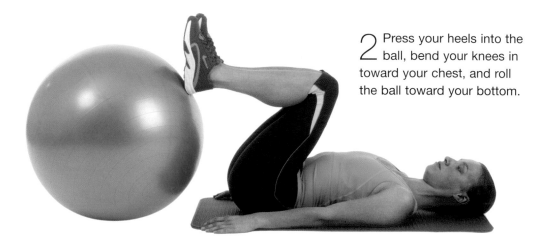

2 Press your heels into the ball, bend your knees in toward your chest, and roll the ball toward your bottom.

3 Extend your legs out to the start position and repeat at least 15 times. Take 2 to 3 seconds to draw the ball in and the same length of time to release the legs.

tips
- Relax your feet so that your calves are not overly involved.
- Use a small ball between your knees if it helps with alignment.
- Regularly check your foot position.

bridge leg curl

moderate

benefits This exercise is a progression of the leg curl. Doing it in a bridge position adds an element of active stabilization, where the torso has to be held in position by strong stabilizers while the limbs move.

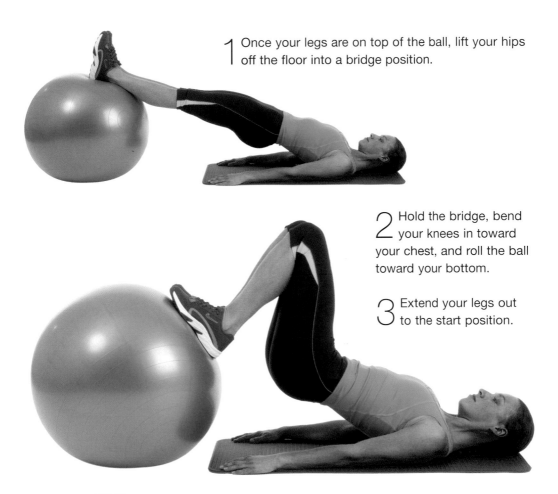

1 Once your legs are on top of the ball, lift your hips off the floor into a bridge position.

2 Hold the bridge, bend your knees in toward your chest, and roll the ball toward your bottom.

3 Extend your legs out to the start position.

tips

■ If you feel your posture going, revert to lying on the floor to finish the repetitions.
■ Make sure that you take your weight across your shoulders and not through your neck or on your head.
■ Try and keep your hips in the same position throughout.

glute stretch

easy

benefits The length of a muscle is as important as its strength. When muscles are worked (during which they contract and shorten). they should always be stretched to try to return them to their pre-work length. This applies as much to the glutes as to all other muscles.

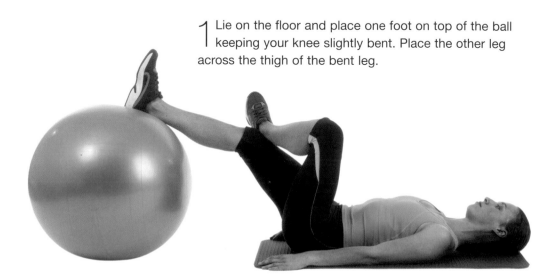

1 Lie on the floor and place one foot on top of the ball keeping your knee slightly bent. Place the other leg across the thigh of the bent leg.

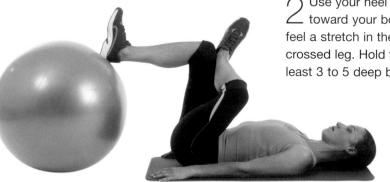

2 Use your heel to roll the ball toward your bottom until you feel a stretch in the hip of the crossed leg. Hold the stretch for at least 3 to 5 deep breaths.

tip

■ Even though your focus is on stretching through the hip, try to keep your core engaged and your shoulders away from your ears.

knee extension

easy

benefits This exercise works to strengthen your quads while at the same time demanding an element of flexibility from your hamstrings. Developing strength and flexibility of opposing muscle groups simultaneously is one of the best and most functional ways to train your body.

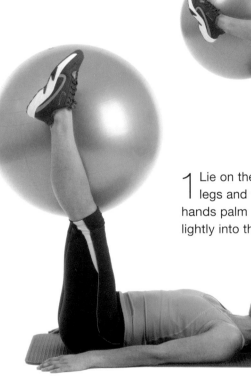

1 Lie on the floor with the ball between your lower legs and feet, knees bent over your hips and your hands palm down on the floor. Press your lower back lightly into the floor and engage your core muscles.

2 Straighten your legs and lift the ball toward the ceiling. Lower back to the start position. Take 2 counts to complete each phase of the movement.

variation

■ Try the same exercise with your palms facing up so that you are unable to assist the leg action by pressing into the floor with your hands.

tips

■ Do not allow momentum to creep in.
■ Keep your knees over your hips at all times to avoid the legs rocking forward as you lift.

shoulder rotator

easy

benefits The rotator cuff muscles of the shoulder allow the arms to turn/twist in and out. Because these muscles are small in relation to other muscles of the body, they are often forgotten when it comes to an exercise program but weak rotators can adversely affect the strength and functioning of the whole shoulder.

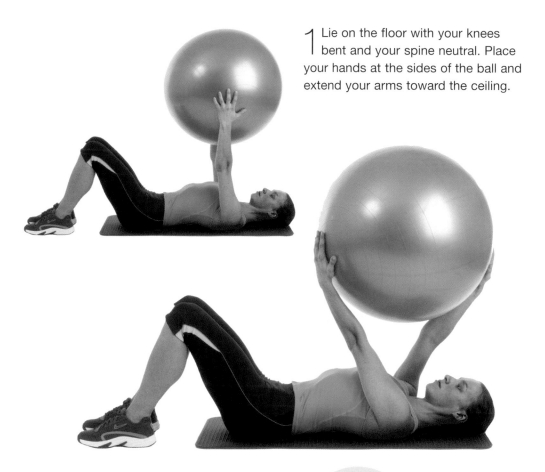

1 Lie on the floor with your knees bent and your spine neutral. Place your hands at the sides of the ball and extend your arms toward the ceiling.

2 Turn the ball so that one hand is at the back of the ball and one at the front. Slowly rotate the ball back to the start position and then turn it in the other direction. Repeat 15 times in each direction.

tips

■ Ease your shoulders toward the floor as you rotate the arms.
■ Do not let your shoulders lift away from the floor.

butterfly stretch

easy

benefits This exercise lengthens and stretches the inner thighs and the internal hip rotator muscles that work to turn the leg in toward the center of the body.

1 Lie on the floor and place both feet high on the front of the ball. Turn your knees out so that the soles of your feet face each other and rest your hands on your knees.

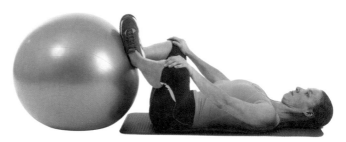

2 Press your feet into the ball and your knees toward the floor until you feel the stretch. Rolling the ball toward your bottom can increase the stretch.

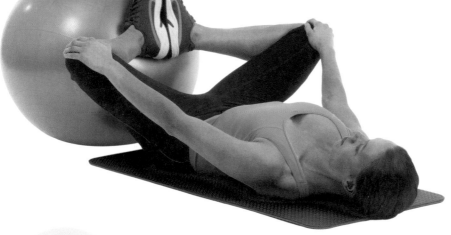

tips

■ Rest your hands on the floor or use them to gently press down on your inner thighs.
■ Try to keep the legs and feet in a symmetrical position.

rotary torso stretch

easy

benefits The oblique muscles, part of the abdominal group, allow rotation of the torso to happen. Like all other muscles, these should be stretched and relaxed after work.

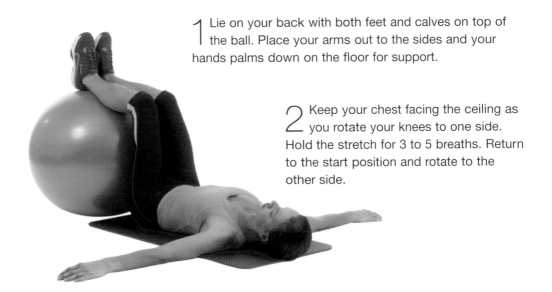

1 Lie on your back with both feet and calves on top of the ball. Place your arms out to the sides and your hands palms down on the floor for support.

2 Keep your chest facing the ceiling as you rotate your knees to one side. Hold the stretch for 3 to 5 breaths. Return to the start position and rotate to the other side.

3 Repeat at least twice to each side. You can use this as a strength exercise if you take only 2 to 3 seconds on each phase and repeat 12 to 15 times to each side.

active calf/hamstring stretch

easy

benefits Any stretching exercise in which muscle groups are combined complements "isolation" stretching in which one muscle group at a time is worked. Compound stretching helps develop a better working relationship between the muscles involved.

1 Lie on the floor with one leg resting on the ball. Place your arms slightly out to the sides and your hands palms down on the floor, to help support your body. Bend the knee of the bent leg so the knee is in line with your hip.

2 Extend the upper leg toward the ceiling and flex the foot of this leg by pointing your toes toward your nose. Ease your leg toward your body by bending at the hip.

tips

■ Keep your hips on the floor.
■ Think about pressing the heel of your extended leg up toward the ceiling. Keep your knee straight.

reverse curl

easy

benefits This exercise strengthens the rectus abdominus or "six pack." Whereas regular abdominal curls work from the top of the abdominals downward, this exercise reverses the initiation of the contraction so that it starts at the lower end of the abdominals and works upward. Working from different ends helps maintain a good balance and comparable levels of strength throughout the length of this muscle.

1 Lie on the floor with the ball hooked against the back of your legs. Place your arms slightly out to the sides and your hands palms down on the floor. Use pressure through your feet and lower legs to press the ball against your thighs. Lightly press your lower back into the floor.

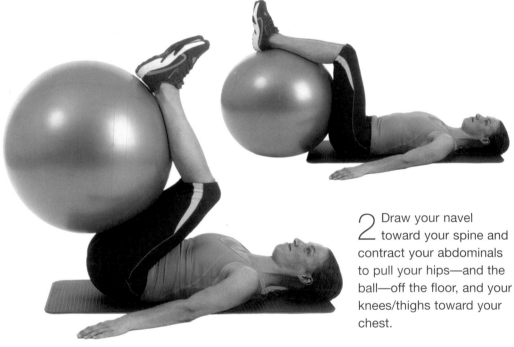

2 Draw your navel toward your spine and contract your abdominals to pull your hips—and the ball—off the floor, and your knees/thighs toward your chest.

tips

■ Keep your shoulders away from your ears and your shoulderblades set down your back.
■ Ensure that all movement is done with good control to make the exercise more effective.

3 Lower your hips and repeat at least 15 times. Take 4 counts to lift and 4 to lower your hips.

leg press

easy

benefits This is a compound exercise that works all the major muscle groups of the legs. This makes it time efficient and good to include in a routine if time is short.

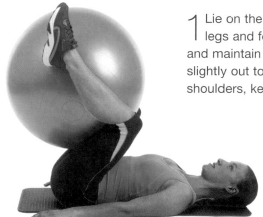

1 Lie on the floor with the ball held between your lower legs and feet. Press your spine lightly into the floor and maintain that pressure throughout. Place your arms slightly out to the sides. Bend your knees toward your shoulders, keeping your hips on the floor.

tip

■ The higher your legs when extended, the easier this exercise is on the abdominals, which have to help stabilize your body. The lower the legs when extended, the harder the abdominals, hip flexors, and quad muscles have to work.

2 Slowly straighten your legs to an angle of 45° to the floor. Return to the start position and repeat at least 15 times. Take 2 counts to extend and the same to bend the knees again.

prone

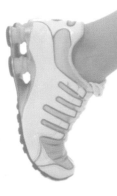

- plank
- lower back stretch
- scapula retraction
- back flye
- calf stretch

- single leg hip extension
- double leg hip extension
- passive quadriceps stretch
- active quadriceps stretch

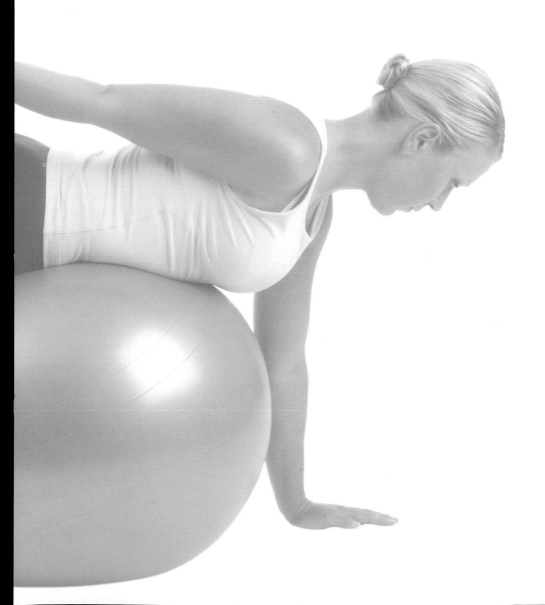

working with the ball in the prone position

Good posture in the "prone" position is just as important as good posture when sitting or standing. There are a few points to remember always, even when your mental focus may be on the movement or exercise.

"Prone" means "face down" and, in relation to the stability ball, you will be face down lying on top of the ball. To try to move from standing to lying on the ball can be difficult. The easiest way to get into a prone position is to roll yourself onto the ball from a kneeling position.

Your head should still be positioned centrally on your shoulders. Avoid tilting your head to the right or left.

Gravity will be felt more on the head in this position and you might find your head and neck dropping forward toward the floor. Your chin should remain off your chest and still be drawn back toward the base of your skull, as it would if you were standing. Your neck should remain in line with the rest of your spine.

Draw your shoulders away from your ears and your shoulderblades down your back, even if your arms are in front of your body, overhead or lifted. Set your core and activate all the muscles involved before you start moving. Also use them when you have to hold the stretches.

Your pelvis should be neutral so that when you set up, your hip bones and pubic bone are like a triangle, set along one plane. Avoid tilting, rocking, or tipping the pelvis unless this is an intentional movement.

Generally your knees and ankles should line up with your hips, whether they are on the floor or suspended in the air. Your legs and feet should be hip-width apart.

Kneel on the floor, knees hip-width apart with the ball in front of you (a). Press the ball lightly against your thighs and bend at your hips and waist to allow your body to fold over the ball. Your chest should come to rest on the top (b). Place your hands on the floor in front of the ball and, lifting your knees off the floor, use your hands and feet to roll yourself forward until the ball is in the required position (c). Once your feet are off the floor, walk your hands forward to change position (d). To return to a kneeling position, walk your hands toward the ball until your feet can touch the ground. Ease your knees to the floor and lift your chest off the ball.

Use this technique to move yourself smoothly onto the ball for all the following exercises.

opposite, top to bottom> **Positioning yourself on the ball to work in the prone position.**

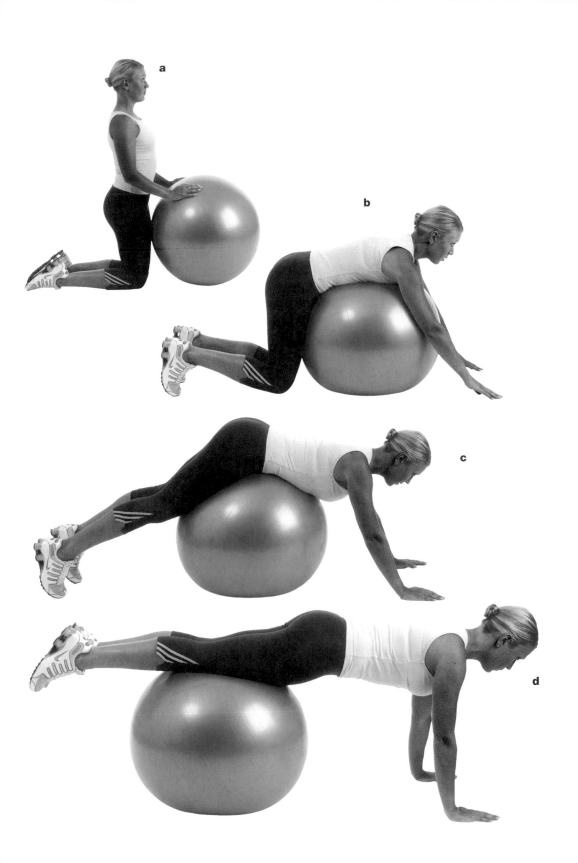

a

b

c

d

jack knife

easy/moderate

benefits This exercise helps improve core stability by strengthening your back and deep abdominals. It also provides a strengthening element for the wrists, arms, and shoulders.

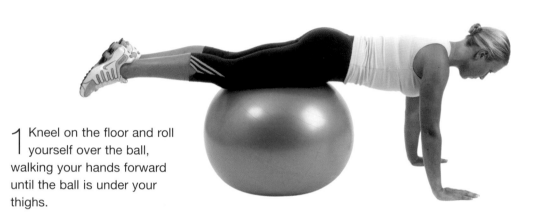

1 Kneel on the floor and roll yourself over the ball, walking your hands forward until the ball is under your thighs.

variation

■ You can make this exercise harder by initially rolling your body forward until the ball is under your shins and your feet are hooked over the ball. As you roll in, lower your knees toward the floor (a). As you roll out, lengthen your legs (b).

a

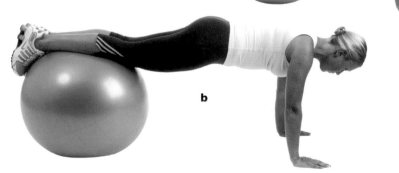

b

2 Draw your navel toward your spine and bend at the hips, using your thighs and knees against the ball to roll it toward your chest. Your hips will lift toward the ceiling and your knees should come in line with your hips. Take 2 to 3 seconds to draw in and the same time to release out for 8 to 12 repetitions. Once you can achieve 12 excellent repetitions, progress to 15.

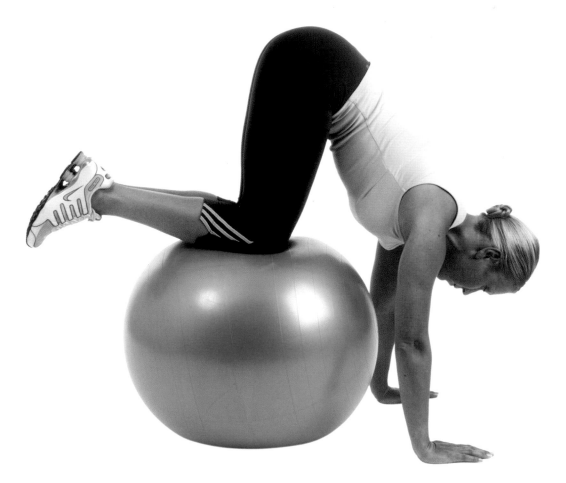

tips

■ Start with a neutral spine and try to maintain it throughout the movement.
■ Make sure that your head stays aligned with the rest of your body and avoid dropping your chin to your chest.

alternating superman

easy/moderate

benefits This exercise strengthens the postural muscles of the back, pelvis, and shoulders as well as working on core stability.

1 To progress the exercise, kneel on the floor, resting your body over the ball with your hands on the floor in front of the ball and your knees and feet hip-width apart.

2 Gently press into the ball as you raise your right leg out behind and your left arm out in front of you. Try to raise them to the same height. Hold the position as still as possible for 10 seconds, then repeat on the other side. Do 8 to 12 repetitions on both sides.

variation

■ Kneel on the floor, resting your body over the ball with your hands on the floor in front of the ball and your knees and feet hip-width apart, then roll yourself forward, lifting your knees off the floor until the ball is under your hips (a).

Raise your right leg out behind and your left arm out in front of you. Try to raise them to the same height (b). Hold the position as still as possible for 10 seconds, then repeat on the other side. Do 8 to 12 repetitions on both sides

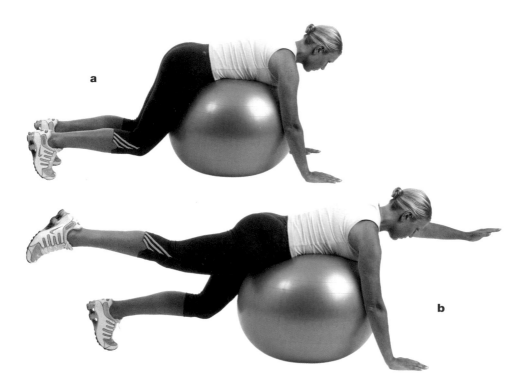

a

b

tips

■ Keep good spinal alignment as you hold and while you move.
■ Remember that your neck is a part of your spine and your head should also be aligned.
■ Keep one foot touching the floor
■ Doing the exercise with knees off the floor can sometimes seem easier because you have more body weight on the ball.

press-up

easy/moderate

benefits This exercise develops upper body strength and stability through the chest, triceps, upper back, arms, and shoulders. It can also help improve core stability.

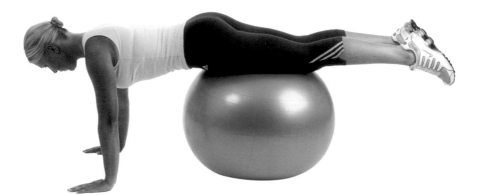

1 Kneel on the floor and roll yourself onto the ball until the ball is under your thighs. Place your hands a little wider than shoulder-width apart with your fingers pointing forward.

2 Keep your spine long as you lower your chest toward the floor, bending your elbows out to the sides.

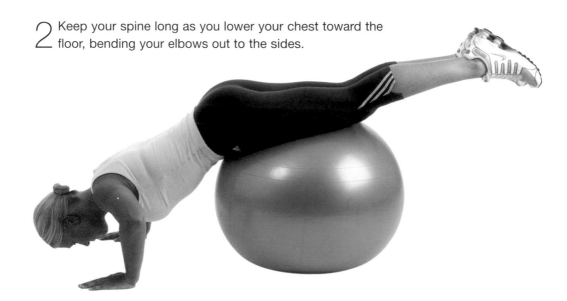

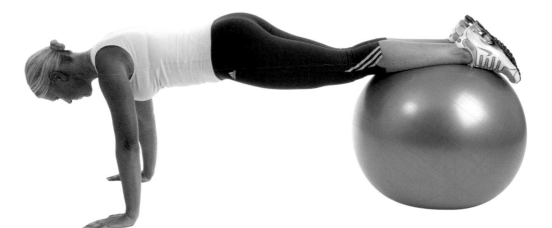

3 Straighten your elbows to press up into the start position. Do 8 to 12 repetitions, taking 2 to 3 seconds to execute each phase of the movement.

tips

■ Maintain a long spine and keep your shoulders away from your ears.
■ You can increase the repetitions as you get stronger.

variation

■ You can make this exercise harder by rolling your body forward so that the ball rests under your shins. You can also focus more on the triceps than the chest by keeping your arms narrow (shoulder-width apart) and having your elbows point backward rather than sideways as you do the press-up.

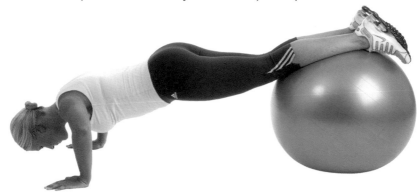

back extension

easy/moderate

benefits This exercise can help strengthen the lower back while at the same time providing a mild stretch for some of the abdominals.

1 Kneel on the floor with your legs hip-width apart and rest your body over the ball. Rest your hands, palms facing up, in the small of your back or place your arms alongside your torso.

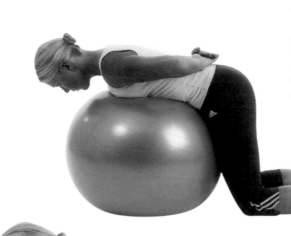

2 Press your pelvis into the ball. Keep your shoulders away from your ears and your shoulderblades pressing down your back as you slowly lift your chest away from the ball. Release your upper body back down. Take about 4 counts to lift and 4 to lower.

variations

■ You can create more of a challenge in this exercise by varying the position of your arms. Have your fingers lightly touch your temples with your elbows pointing straight out to the sides (a).

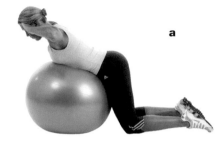

a

■ Or do the exercise with one or both arms extended out in front of you, trying to keep the inner arm in line with your ears (b).

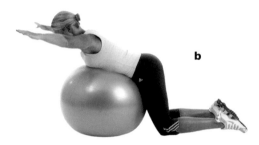

b

■ You can also make more stability demands of the body by lifting your knees off the floor, keeping your feet hip-width apart. You can then do all of the arm variations in this position (c).

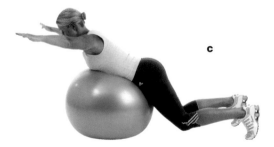

c

■ If you initially find it difficult to stay still on the ball in position (c), rest your feet against a wall and this will help you stabilize (d, e).

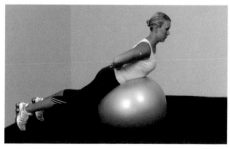

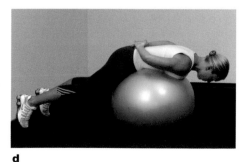

d

e

upper back stretch

easy

benefits This exercise releases tension and stress from the upper back and stretches and relaxes the muscles in this area.

1 Kneel on the floor and rest your body over the ball. Allow your shoulderblades to move apart and your arms to rest on the floor in front of the ball. Let the ball take your weight. Hold the position for at least 3 to 5 deep breaths.

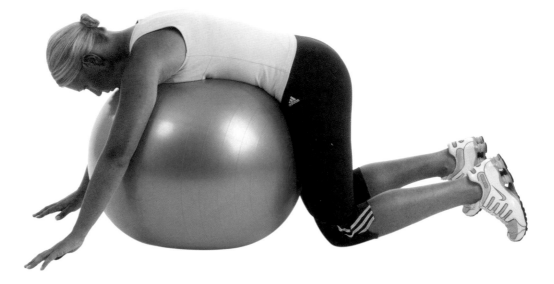

tip

■ Close your eyes and focus on the pace and depth of your breathing.

plank

easy/moderate

benefits This exercise trains the body to activate the deep abdominal, back, and pelvic floor muscles at the same time. It improves core stability and internal strength and provides a strength challenge for the upper body and torso.

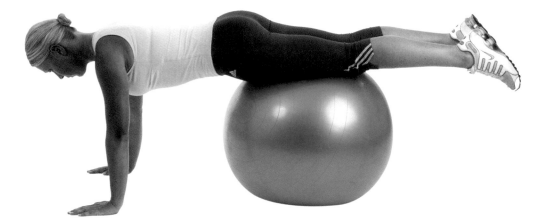

variations

■ To progress this exercise, first have the ball under your shins (a) then have your toes (b) resting on top of the ball.

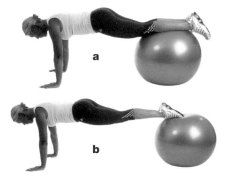

■ With any of these positions you could lift one leg/foot off the ball and challenge the body to stabilize so that neither the ball nor the body moves.

1 Roll onto your ball from a kneeling position and walk your hands forward until the ball is under your thighs. Draw you stomach in and your navel toward your spine, and set your pelvis in neutral. Hold the position for up to 10 seconds then walk the hands back, coming onto your knees to rest. Repeat 8 to 12 times.

tips

■ If your wrists hurt or become uncomfortable, make a fist and rest on your knuckles instead or have some dumbbells in your hands and allow these to rest on the floor.
■ Try to keep the body in neutral alignment as you hold the position.

lower back stretch

easy

benefits This exercise releases tension and stress from the lower back and stretches and relaxes the muscles in this area.

1 Roll yourself onto the ball from a kneeling position until the ball is under your waist and your forearms rest on the floor. Have your toes lightly touching the floor. Allow the ball to take your weight until there is no tension in the lower back. Hold the position for at least 3 to 5 deep breaths.

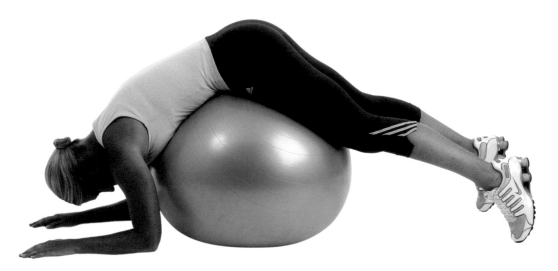

tip

■ Close your eyes and focus on the pace and depth of your breathing.

scapula retraction

easy

benefits This exercise helps strengthen the upper back and improves its ability to stabilize. It will often also improve posture as it works to reverse the commonly seen rounded shoulder syndrome.

1 Kneel on the floor and rest your chest on the ball allowing your arms to rest at the sides with your fingers touching the floor.

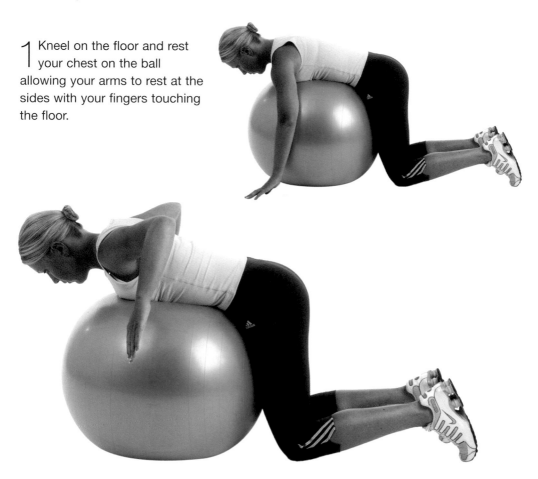

2 Press your chest into the ball. Slowly squeeze your shoulderblades together and then release. Do 8 to 12 repetitions, taking 2 to 3 seconds on each phase.

tip

■ Focus on moving your shoulderblades rather than your shoulders or elbows.

back flye

easy

benefits This exercise strengthens the muscles of the upper back, including the back of the shoulders.

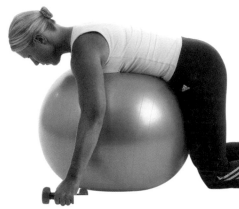

1 Place a light handweight on either side of your ball—start with about 4½ lb (2 kg). Set yourself up draped over the ball with your knees and feet on the floor and then pick up the weights.

2 Keep your elbows slightly bent and gently squeeze your shoulderblades together as you lift your arms out to the sides. Release to the start position and repeat up to 12 times. Take 2 to 3 seconds to execute each phase of the movement.

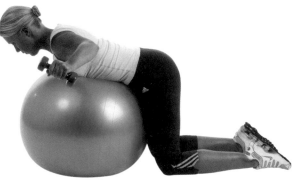

tips

■ Keep your shoulders down, away from your ears.
■ If you are not used to working with weights, practice without first to make sure that you get the technique right. You should feel the contraction at the back of the shoulders and between the shoulderblades.
■ You can increase the weight of the dumbbells as you grow stronger.

variation

■ To progress this exercise, lift your knees off the floor.

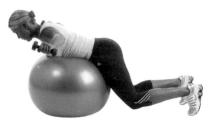

calf stretch

easy

benefits This exercise lengthens the calf muscles.

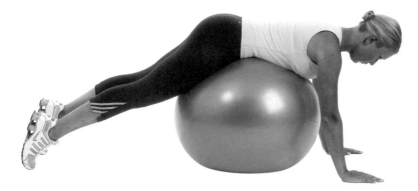

1 Rest your body over the ball with your hands on the floor in front of you for support. Your heels should be lifted, your toes should be on the floor, and the ball should be under your hips.

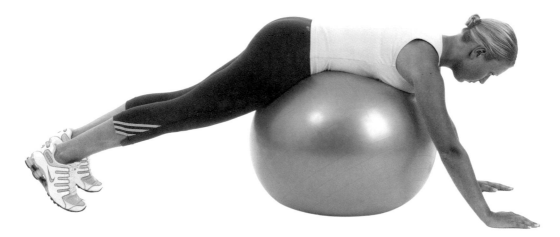

2 Roll the ball back and gently press your heels toward the floor without moving the position of your hands. Hold the stretch for at least 3 to 5 deep breaths. Release and repeat if you feel your calves need more of a stretch.

tip

■ If you feel your muscles release a little and your heels are not yet touching the floor, try to develop the stretch by easing your heels slightly closer to the floor.

single leg hip extension

easy

benefits This exercise strengthens the glutes and lengthens the hip flexors.

1 Lie on the ball with your legs straight out behind you and your toes touching the floor. The ball should be under your waist and hips. Place your hands on the floor in front of you.

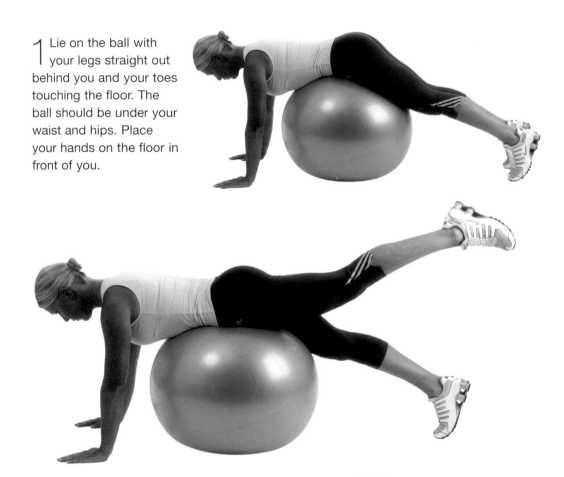

2 Keep your hips pressed into the ball as you lift one leg and straighten your hip joint. Lift and lower the same leg 12 times, taking 2 counts on each phase, and then change sides. You can lift the legs alternately, which will give one leg a little rest while the other works.

tips

■ The higher you are on the ball, the smaller the range of movement you will have.

■ Having your knee bent gives you a greater range of movement. Lifting a straight leg will mean a smaller range.

double leg hip extension

moderate

benefits This exercise requires greater strength than lifting one leg. There is also a benefit from working synergistic muscles simultaneously.

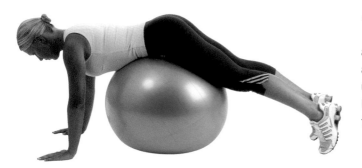

1 Lie on the ball with your toes touching the floor and your legs hip-width apart. The ball should be under your waist and hips. Place your hands on the floor in front of you.

2 Press your hips into the ball as you lift both legs. Your elbows may bend slightly. Lift and lower your legs up to 12 times, taking 2 counts on each phase of the movement.

tips

■ Think about stabilizing your core and check that your shoulders have not drifted toward your ears.

passive quadriceps stretch

easy

benefits This exercise lengthens the quads, the muscles that cross the hip joint and run down the front of the thighs.

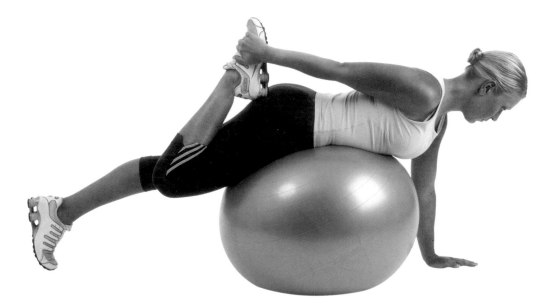

1 Lie on the ball with your toes touching the floor and your legs hip-width apart. The ball should be under your waist and hips and your hands on the floor in front of you.

2 Lift your right leg, bend your knee, and, grasping your ankle with your right hand, ease your heel toward your bottom, keeping your left hand on the floor. Hold the stretch for at least 3 to 5 deep breaths. Repeat on the other side.

tips

■ Watch the position of your head in this unsupported position.
■ Ensure that your shoulders are parallel and you have not shortened your body on the side of the stretching leg.

active quadriceps stretch

moderate

benefits This stretch helps lengthen the quad muscles in the front of the thighs. It is called an "active" stretch because the muscles of your hamstrings have to hold your leg in place without assistance (for example, from your hand holding your ankle), as happens in a "passive" stretch. As an "active" stretch it also addresses the working synergy between opposing muscle groups, in this case, hamstrings and quadriceps.

tip

■ Ensure that your hips stay parallel and that the hip of the lifting leg does not start to turn out to the side.

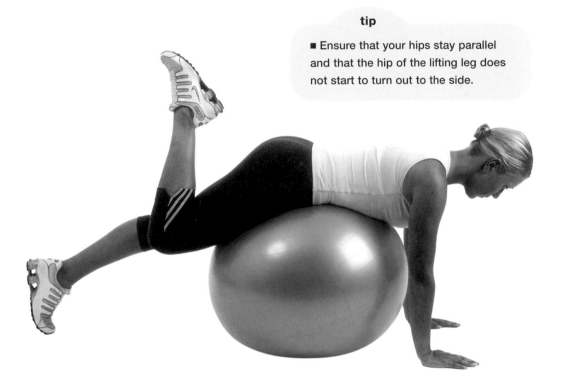

1 Lie on the ball with your toes touching the floor and your legs hip-width apart. The ball should be under your waist and hips and your hands on the floor in front of you.

2 Gently press both hip bones into the ball and lift one leg, bending your knee to bring your heel toward your bottom. Hold the stretch for at least 3 to 5 deep breaths. Repeat on the other side.

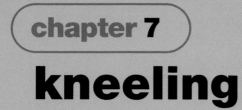

chapter 7

kneeling

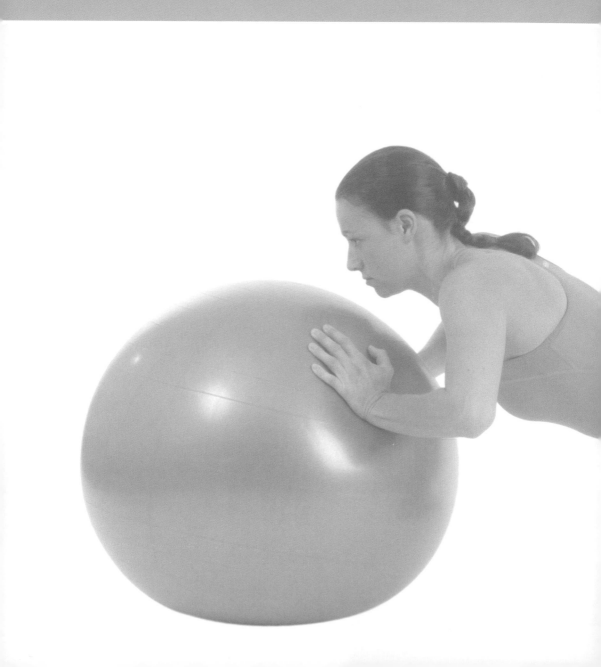

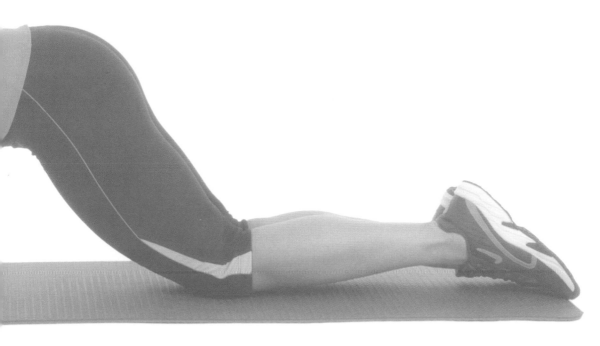

working with the ball in a kneeling position

The only postural change in this position is in the knee joint and lower leg. The knee joint is bent and the ankles and feet should line up with the knees. All the previous postural cues mentioned in the Standing chapter apply.

Whenever you are on "all fours" or kneeling up, check that your knees are hip-width apart. On "all fours" your spine should be long and extended with a natural curve in your lower back. Your pelvic floor should be engaged and your deep abdominals drawn in toward your spine to help support your lower back. Your pelvis should be aligned and fixed. Check your head and neck position.

Remember to have a mat or a towel to place under your knees for cushioning and comfort if you are working on a hard surface. Make sure that it is not so thick that it affects your balance as you kneel.

We don't often think about the effect of gravity on the body as we go about our daily lives because we know no other state. However, gravity is a substantial external force that constantly applies pressure to the body. When we are on "all fours," as in the kneeling position used for this group of exercises, gravity is pressing down on the head, neck, and spine. If the core muscles are not activated to help attain good alignment and if they do not have the strength to then maintain that position, sometimes, as parts of the body move, problems with posture may occur that will affect the safety of the exercise.

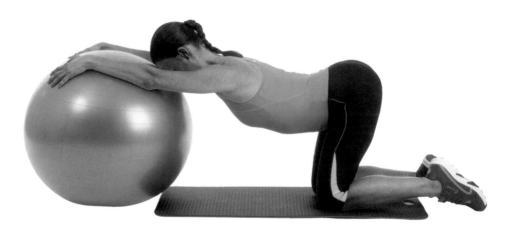

above> **Often when people work in the kneeling position, they do not activate the core muscles, which means their back sags toward the floor, as shown here. The transverse abdominus and the pelvic floor muscles must be activated to help support the lower back.**

lat stretch

easy

benefits This exercise stretches and lengthens the latissimus dorsi, the muscles just under the shoulderblades that work to pull the elbows down toward the hips.

1 Kneel on the floor with your legs and feet hip-width apart and your hands and forearms on the ball in front of you. Engage your core muscles, bend forward at your hips and roll the ball forward with your hands until you feel a stretch in your lats. Your hips should be in line with your knees.

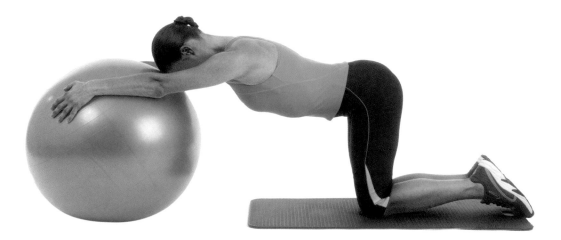

2 Hold the position for at least 3 to 5 deep breaths and then roll the ball back toward you, lifting your chest.

3 Repeat the sequence 3 or 4 times depending on how tight your lats are or you can simply hold the position for longer.

tips

■ Think about drawing your shoulders and shoulderblades away from your head as you hold the position.
■ Check that you are not sagging in your mid section (stomach and lower back).

upper back stretch

easy

benefits This position releases tension across the upper back.

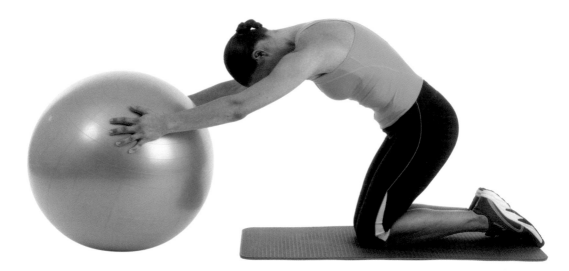

1 Place your hands at the sides of the ball and bend forward slightly from your hips. Tuck your chin in toward your chest and draw your chest away from the ball, separating your shoulderblades and rounding your upper back as you do so. You should feel a stretch across your upper back.

2 Hold the position for 3 to 5 deep breaths and repeat if you feel your back needs more of a stretch.

tip

■ Use the ball as an anchor point that you can pull away from, so try to keep the ball on one spot and move your body into the stretch.

quadriceps stretch

moderate

benefits This position stretches and lengthens the muscles in the front of the thighs.

1 Kneel on the floor in a lunge position. Lean forward to rest the front of your back foot against the ball. You may support yourself with your hands on the floor as you do this. Use one hand to stabilize the ball if necessary and place the other on your front thigh as you lengthen your spine and gently tuck your hips under until you feel a stretch in your hip joint and the front of your thigh.

tip

 If balancing is difficult do this exercise in front of a wall or have something stable beside you that you can lightly hold onto. Your challenge will then be to improve your balance in this position so that you no longer need the external assistance.

2 Hold the position while you breathe in 3 to 5 deep breaths. Repeat on the other side.

chest stretch

easy

benefits In people who have bad posture, including rounded shoulders, the chest muscles will usually be tight and shortened. This is part of the reason why the shoulders tend to round. Stretching the chest will lengthen the muscles and assist in a return to good posture.

1 Kneel on all fours with the ball just off to the right side. Ensure that your hips are over your knees.

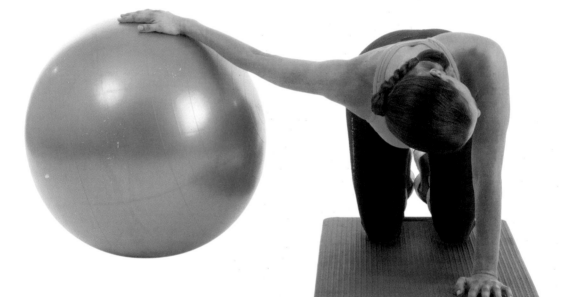

2 Place your right hand on top of the ball, turn your head to the left, and roll the ball away from you to the right until you feel a stretch in the front of the shoulder and chest. Hold for at least 3 to 5 breaths and repeat on the other side.

tips

■ Keep your torso strong to avoid sagging in your mid section.
■ Do not allow your hips to twist.

press-up

easy

benefits A press-up is a compound movement that, if done properly, encourages the muscles of the upper body and torso to work together effectively and efficiently. Compound exercises promote better synergy between different muscle groups.

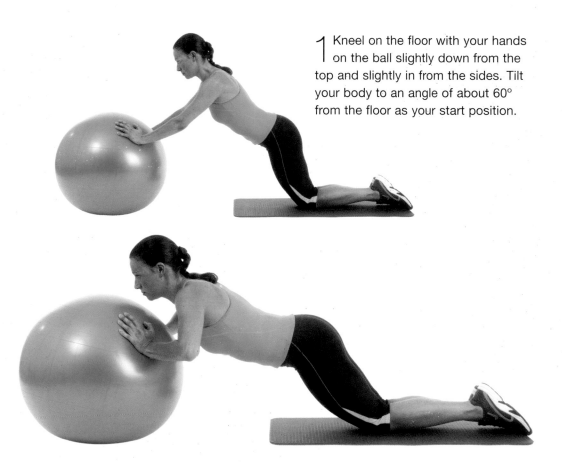

1 Kneel on the floor with your hands on the ball slightly down from the top and slightly in from the sides. Tilt your body to an angle of about 60° from the floor as your start position.

2 Stabilize your torso and bend your elbows out to the sides as you lower your chest toward the ball. Push your body away from the ball by straightening your arms to return to the start position.

tips

■ Lower your whole body as a unit.
■ Check that your neck stays aligned with the rest of your spine and that your head and chin do not dip toward your chest as you move.

ball roll

easy/moderate

benefits This exercise will help strengthen the muscles of the upper and middle back as well as involve the core stability muscles.

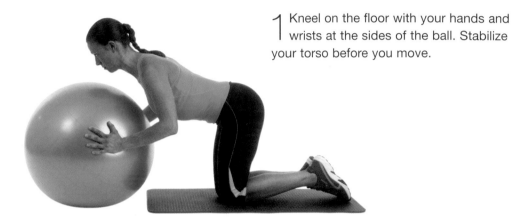

1 Kneel on the floor with your hands and wrists at the sides of the ball. Stabilize your torso before you move.

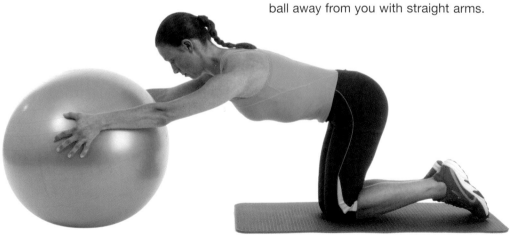

2 Keeping your hips over your knees, bend forward at the hips, and roll the ball away from you with straight arms.

3 Return to the start position by rolling the ball toward you, still keeping your arms straight. Repeat this exercise up to 15 times.

variations

■ You can intensify the movement
by keeping your hips straighter
and leaning forward from your
knees as you roll the ball. Work on
keeping your hips straight as you
lower and lift.

tips

■ Your torso should remain stabilized throughout the
movement.
■ Pay particular attention to the position of your shoulders.
■ Press your arms into the ball as you roll.

chapter 8
side-lying

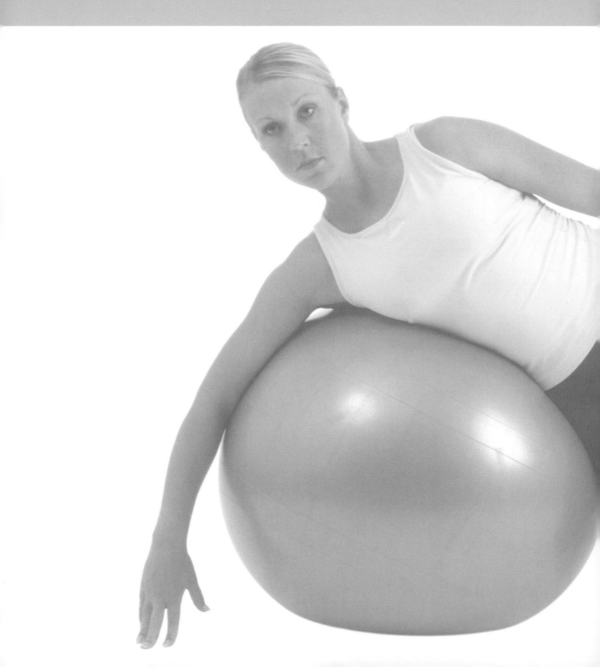

- lateral torso flexion/extension
- hip abduction (floor)
- hip abduction (ball)
- hip adduction (floor)
- hip adduction (ball)
- glute stretch
- neck stretch

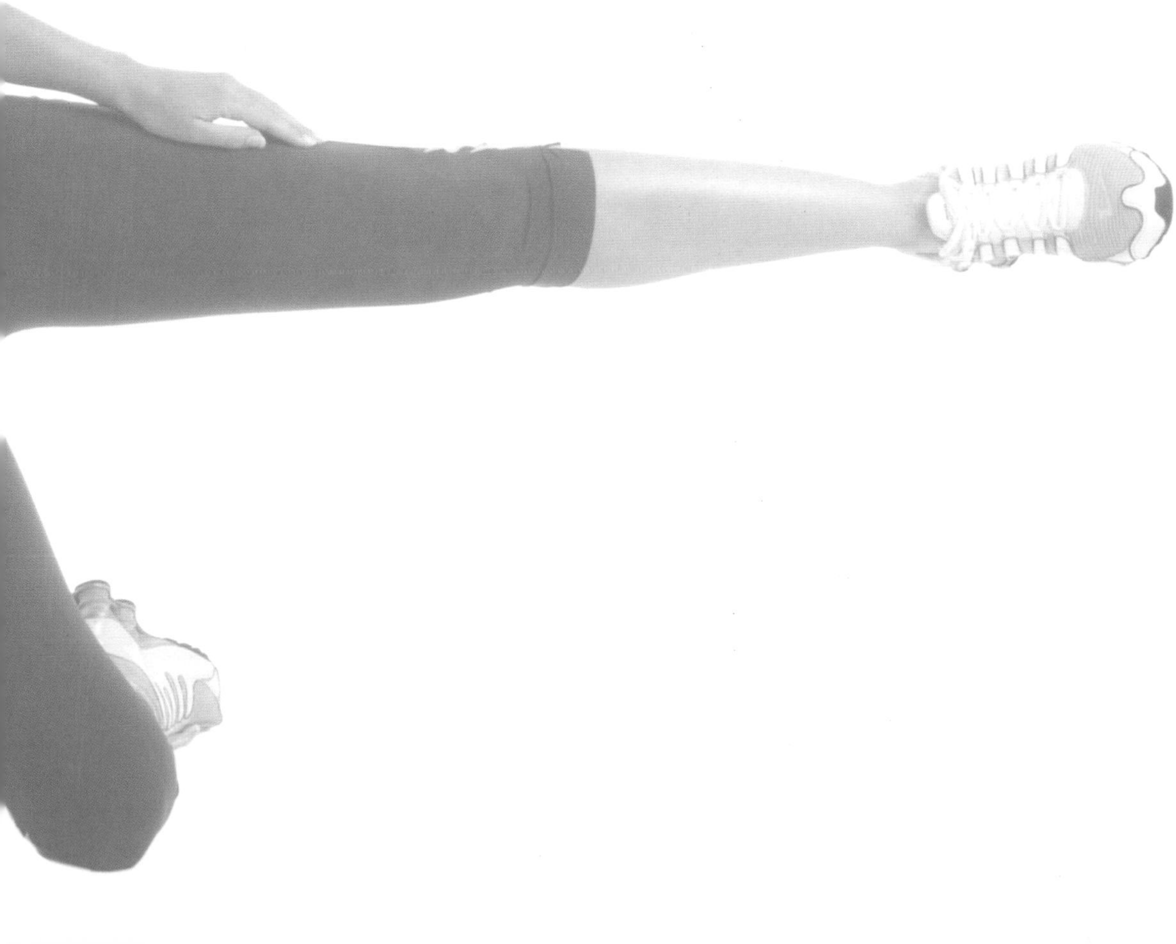

working with the ball in a side-lying position

The postural positioning is just as important in this position, which is more unilateral in that you work on one side and then the other, as it is in the positions where both sides or opposing sides work together. Because you have less surface area of the body on the ball than when lying prone or supine, these exercises are likely to feel more difficult and the balance aspects be more of a challenge.

Watch for your top hip rolling forward or backward as the body works in this position. Try to stabilize yourself internally so that movement of the body and the ball are kept to a minimum. Always establish neutral posture before you start to move. The only time you will not be in neutral is during the neck and torso stretches when your body is required to curve itself over the ball.

Moving onto the ball should be done carefully. Use your hands and feet as much as is necessary to help support your body as you get on and off the ball. Have a towel or mat as cushioning for your knees.

Kneel on the floor with the ball beside you (a). Lightly press the ball into the side of your thigh and then roll the ball away from you along the side of the body, always keeping the connection between the side of the body and the ball. As the ball rolls up the side of the body, bring it to a stop in the required position (b). You will then be able to lift your body onto the ball by extending your legs (c). To change your position on the ball, walk your feet toward the ball so that the ball will roll farther down your body (d); walk your feet away from the ball and it will roll up toward your armpit.

Come off the ball by reversing the actions you took to get on.

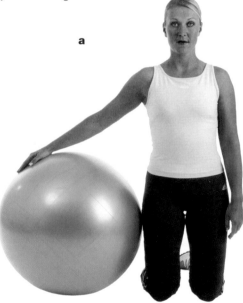

a

above and opposite, top to bottom> **Positioning yourself on the ball to work in a side-lying position.**

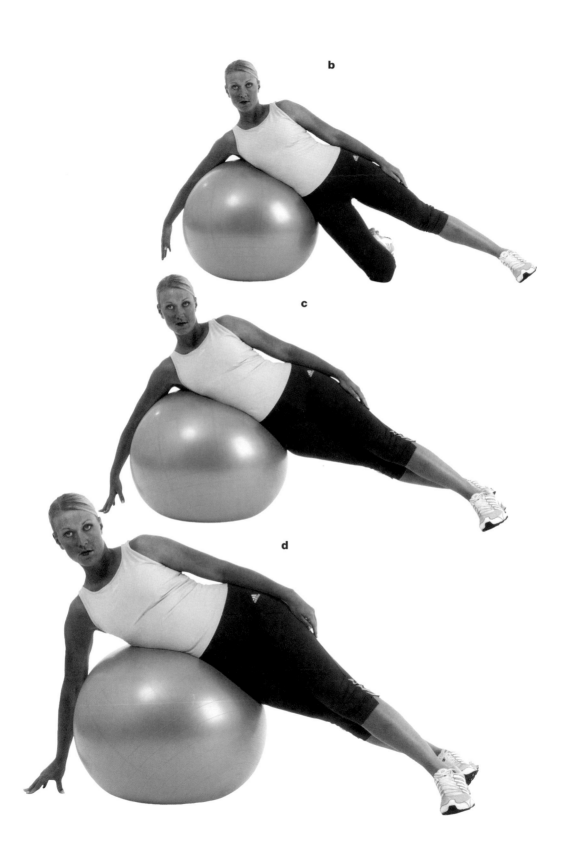

b

c

d

lateral torso flexion/extension

easy/moderate

benefits This exercise strengthens the oblique abdominals and stabilizing muscles.

1 Kneel on the floor with the ball beside you. Lower yourself onto the ball so that your waist, ribs, and armpit rest against it. Straighten your top leg to give additional support. Place your bottom hand against your temple so that your elbow points out to the side and place your top hand on the ball.

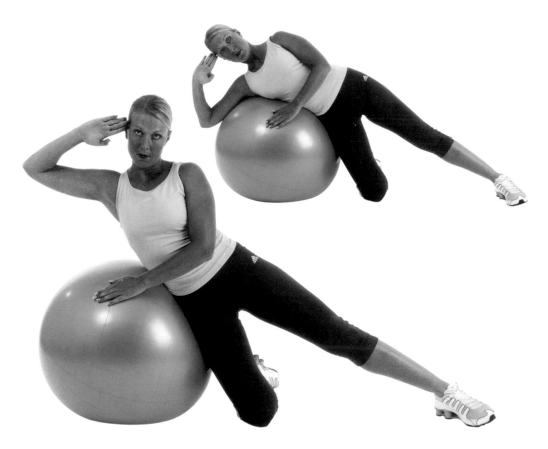

2 Lift your armpit and upper ribs away from the ball while keeping your lower ribs and hip pressing into the ball. Gently release back to the start position.

3 Do 12 to 15 repetitions, taking 2 counts to lift and 2 to lower. Repeat on the other side.

tips

■ Engage your core muscles to help keep you strong and still, other than for the part of the body you are intentionally moving.
■ Avoid your hips rolling forward or back.

variations

■ You can increase the workload by changing arm and leg position, by placing both hands at your temples, or by straightening both legs and staggering them, with one arm or both arms lifting (a, b).

■ If you find it difficult to balance when you straighten your legs, place your feet against a wall (c, d). Take yourself away from the wall as your balance gets better.

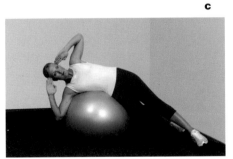

c

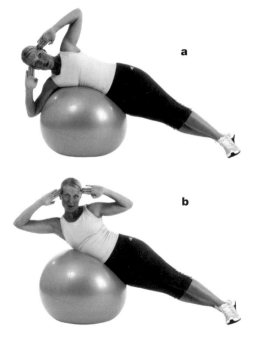

a

b

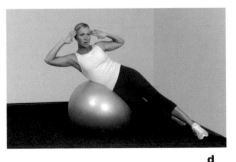

d

hip abduction (floor)

easy

benefits This exercise strengthens the abductors, the outer thigh muscles that work to lift the leg away from the midline of the body.

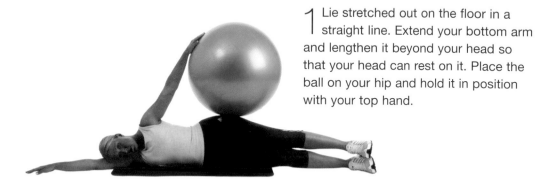

1 Lie stretched out on the floor in a straight line. Extend your bottom arm and lengthen it beyond your head so that your head can rest on it. Place the ball on your hip and hold it in position with your top hand.

2 Engage your pelvic floor muscles and draw your navel to your spine, keeping your spine neutral. Gently lift your top leg and roll the ball toward your knees. Add a little more resistance by pressing the ball into your leg as you lift.

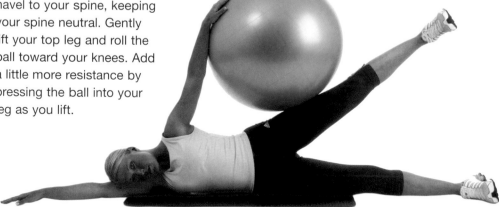

3 Repeat 12 to 15 times. Start by taking 4 counts on each phase and then reduce it to 2 counts for more of a challenge. Progress to the quicker movement only when you can maintain good control and technique.

tips

■ Ensure that your hips do not rock forward or backward.
■ As you lift your leg check that your knee and toes face forward and do not turn toward the ceiling.

hip abduction (ball)

easy/moderate

benefits This exercise strengthens the abductors that work to lift the leg away from the midline of the body. Using a ball works more effectively on core stability than doing the exercise without a ball. This exercise also improves the synergy of different muscle groups working together.

1 Lie sideways on the ball with the knee of your bottom leg on the floor and your top leg straight. Place your bottom hand on the floor for support and your top hand on the ball or resting against your top thigh.

2 Lift and lower your top leg 12 to 15 times, taking 4 counts for each phase of the movement.

tip

■ Check that your top shoulder has not rolled forward. Setting your shoulders and shoulderblades down will help prevent this.

variation

■ The progression of this exercise is to have both legs straight and stacked one above the other. Balance the body and lift the top leg.

hip adduction (floor)

easy

benefits This exercise strengthens the adductors, the inner thigh muscles that work to bring the legs together. It is easier to start this exercise on the floor and then progress to the ball.

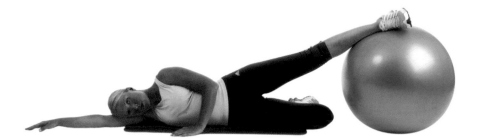

1 Lie on the floor in a straight line with your bottom arm extended beyond your head and your head resting on it. Your other hand can rest on the floor for support or along your top thigh. Place your top foot on the ball and bend the knee of your bottom leg to 90°.

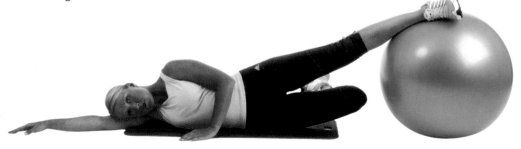

2 Lift and lower your bottom leg 12 to 15 times, taking 4 counts for each phase of the movement.

tip

■ Ensure that your top shoulder and your hips do not rock out of position.

3 You may cut the timing of the movement to 2 counts on each phase when you can lift the leg and still maintain good position.

hip adduction (ball)

moderate

benefits This exercise strengthens the inner thigh muscles that work to bring the legs together. Done on the ball, it also improves core stability and the synergy of different muscle groups working together.

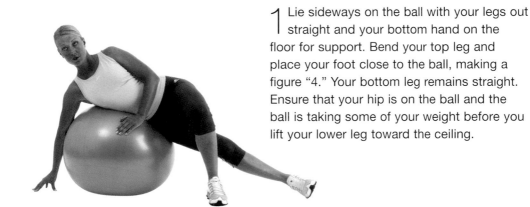

1 Lie sideways on the ball with your legs out straight and your bottom hand on the floor for support. Bend your top leg and place your foot close to the ball, making a figure "4." Your bottom leg remains straight. Ensure that your hip is on the ball and the ball is taking some of your weight before you lift your lower leg toward the ceiling.

2 Lift and lower your bottom leg 12 to 15 times, taking 4 counts for each phase of the movement. You may cut the timing of the movement to 2 counts on each phase when you can lift the leg and still maintain good position.

tips

■ The farther onto the ball you are, the easier it is to lift the leg.
■ Stabilize your torso to avoid movement of the ball and your body.

glute stretch

easy

benefits This exercise lengthens and stretches the glutes and the "external rotators." You may also feel a stretch in the outer thigh muscles of the lower leg.

1 Kneel on the floor with the ball beside you and lie into the ball so that it rests against your ribs and waist. Place your hands around the ball to give support to your body.

2 Lift yourself onto the ball and straighten your bottom leg. Cross your top leg over to make a figure "4." Place the foot of the bottom leg as close to the ball as you can and press your hips into the ball. Let your hips drop toward the floor until you feel a stretch in the hip and thigh of your bottom leg.

3 Use your top hand to ease the knee of your crossed leg toward the ball until you feel a stretch in the top hip.

tip

■ One person may feel these stretches slightly differently and more or less intensely than another person depending on how tight or not they are within each muscle group.

neck stretch

easy

benefits This exercise eases tension in the area of the neck and upper back. It also helps to lengthen the neck by having the shoulder ease away from the ear.

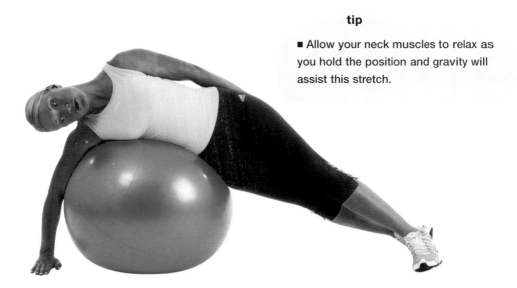

tip

■ Allow your neck muscles to relax as you hold the position and gravity will assist this stretch.

1 Lie sideways on the ball with your feet staggered (top foot in front of your bottom foot) and your hand on the floor. Draw your shoulders away from your ears and your shoulderblades toward your waist. Rest your top arm on your thigh or place it just behind your back. Tilt your head toward the floor, opening out the upper side of your neck. Stabilize through the torso to help keep the ball still and torso movement to a minimum.

2 Hold the position for at least 3 to 5 deep breaths. Release and repeat on the other side.

variation

■ For a torso stretch, lie sideways on the ball with your feet staggered (top foot in front of your bottom foot) and your hand on the floor. Press your body into the ball and slowly lift your top arm overhead until you feel a stretch along the upper side of your body. Hold for 3 to 5 breaths and repeat on the other side.

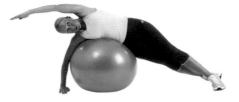

programs

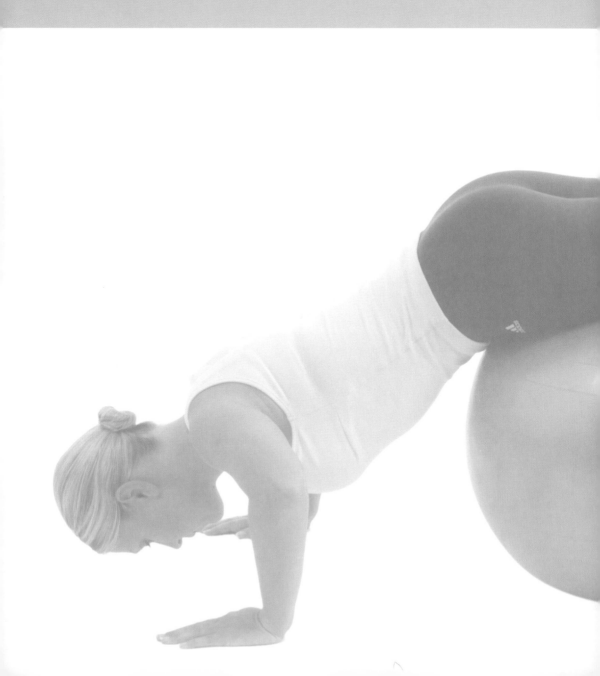

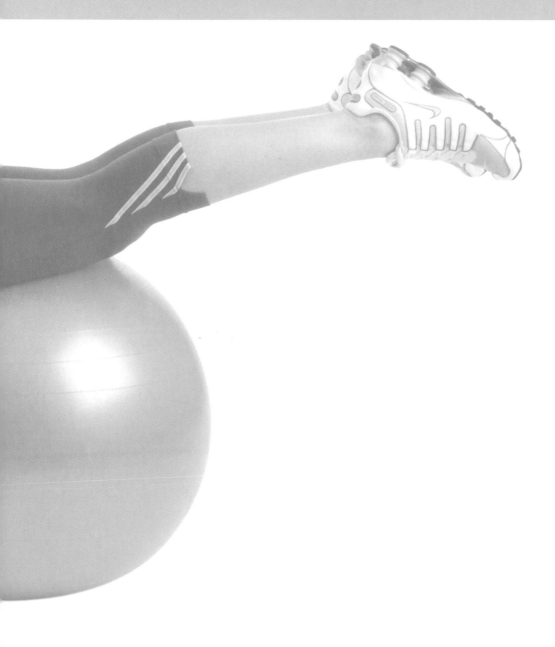

- overall body strength sequence
- overall body flexibility sequence
- core/torso stabilization sequence
- upper body sequence
- lower body sequence

overall body strength sequence

Muscle strength, or muscle tone, is vital. If your muscles are not strong enough to lift and move your bones or hold your bones in place, function is affected. Muscle strength is normally trained by using heavy resistance or weight and doing a small number of repetitions.

Muscular endurance is the ability of the muscle to overcome a resistance or to sustain a contraction for an extended period of time. This is normally trained by doing a greater number of repetitions while lifting less weight.

Most of the exercises on the ball use body weight as the resistance you work with, in addition to more or less resistance from gravity, depending on the body position. The advantage of using a ball rather than a machine is that in many exercises you have to balance on the ball in order to be able to do the exercise, which creates another layer of fitness that involves your posture, alignment, and core stability. It demands strength from the inside, affects the way you do the exercise, and relates to the quality and technique of your movement. This is a foundational element of training that has been ignored for years.

Always finish your strength workout with some focused stretching.

1 hour

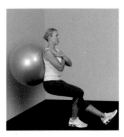

Single leg squat
against the wall
(see page 29)

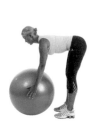

Moving hip hinge
(see page 32)

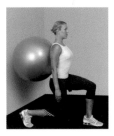

Lunge against
the wall
(see page 30)

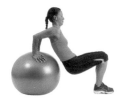

Seated walk
(see page 57)

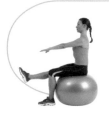

Opposition arm to leg
balance
(see page 53)

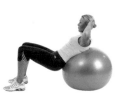

Incline abdominal curl
(see page 73)

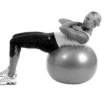

Oblique curl
(see page 74)

Triceps dip (moderate)
(see page 69)

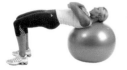

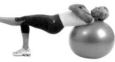

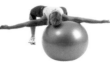

Bridge
(see page 75)

Bridge single leg
balance
(see page 76)

Lateral roll
(see page 82)

Jack knife
(see page 104)

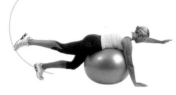

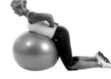

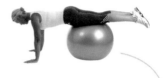

Alternating superman
(see page 106)

Back extension
(see page 110)

Plank
(see page 113)

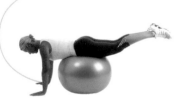

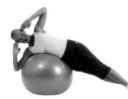

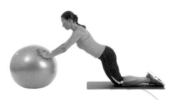

Double leg hip extension
(see page 119)

Lateral torso flexion/extension
(see page 136)

Press-up
(see page 129)

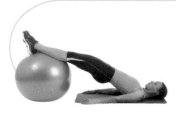

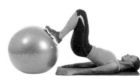

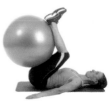

Hip extension
(see page 89)

Leg curl
(see page 90)

Reverse curl
(see page 98)

overall body flexibility sequence

Flexibility is the ability to use muscles to take a joint through its potential full range of movement. There are "normal ranges" of flexibility that healthy adult joints should be able to work through. If you have strength but lack flexibility this can restrict movement. If you have flexibility but lack strength, this affects the integrity of your joints. In both situations, there is a resultant increase in the risk of injury. Developing flexibility involves the lengthening or stretching of muscles.

Flexibility work is best done when the body is warm because the warmer the muscles are, the more pliable they will be. This is generally why stretching is usually left to the end of workouts. But as long as the body is warmed up, you can stretch a muscle group or body section immediately after you have worked it and before you go on to work the next section or muscle group. It does not have to be left to the end.

Although in many exercise situations strength and flexibility are dealt with separately, in reality they affect one another and should be developed together.

The following is a stretch sequence, but you can use any of these exercises after a workout or intersperse them between different strength focused exercises.

1 hour

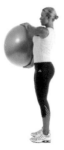 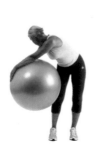 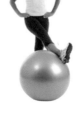 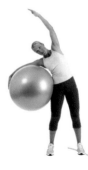

Shoulder stretch	Rotary torso stretch	Hip abductor stretch	Lateral torso stretch
(see page 36)	**(see page 39)**	**(see page 44)**	**(see page 40)**

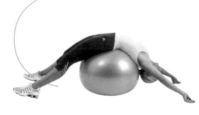 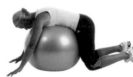 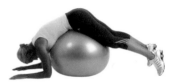

Abdominal stretch	Upper back stretch	Lower back stretch
(see page 78)	**(see page 112)**	**(see page 114)**

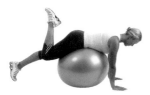

Active quad stretch
(see page 121)

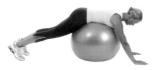

Calf stretch
(see page 117)

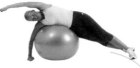

Torso stretch
(see page 143)

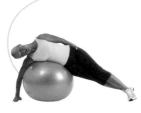

Neck stretch
(see page 143)

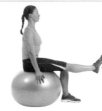

Active hamstring
stretch
(see page 55)

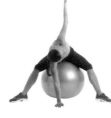

Adductor triangle
stretch
(see page 61)

Hip flexor stretch
with tibialis
(see page 63)

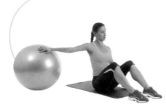

Single arm chest stretch
(see page 66)

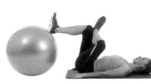

Glute stretch
(see page 92)

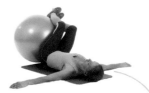

Rotary torso stretch
(see page 96)

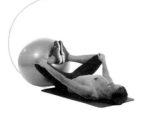

Butterfly stretch
(see page 95)

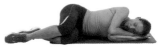

Wind down—full body stretch
(see page 19)

Wind down—fetal position
(see page 19)

core/torso stabilization sequence

We have already spoken about the importance of the core and of stabilizing it when you exercise. It is now known that movement of the limbs affects the core so the strength or lack of strength in the core affects the limbs. Sometimes it is hard to believe that the two are connected but if you stand up and place your right hand behind your back, press your fingers hard into the muscle just to the right of your lower spine, then lift your left arm above your head, you should feel movement in the muscles under your fingers as you lift.

As stated earlier, most of the exercises in this book will tax the core and torso muscles. The following sequence will help a) the upper and lower body work effectively together; b) the front of the body to co-ordinate with the back; c) the right and left sides to work in a symmetrical and co-ordinated fashion; d) the torso to maintain balanced and stable support for the action of other body parts; e) the torso to actively internally stabilize itself during daily activities in a safe, protective position without external support; and f) the upper and lower body to co-ordinate with the torso. It is important that neither upper nor lower body are over- or underdeveloped and that they can move through a large range of motion in many directions with active flexibility and usable, functional strength.

1 hour

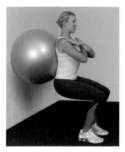

Squat against
the wall
(see page 28)

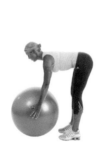

Moving hip hinge
(see page 32)

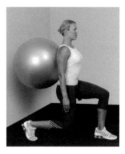

Lunge against
the wall
(see page 30)

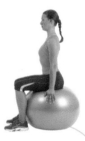

Pelvic tilt
(see page 49)

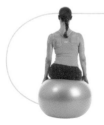

Lateral pelvic tilt
(see page 50)

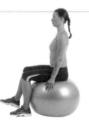

Single leg balance
(see page 51)

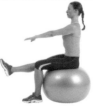

Opposition arm to leg
balance
(see page 53)

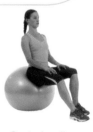

Seated walk
(see page 57)

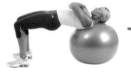

Bridge
(see page 75)

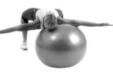

Lateral roll
(see page 82)

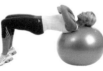

Heel raise
(see page 84)

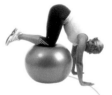

Jack knife
(see page 104)

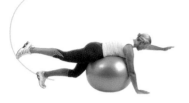

Alternating superman
(see page 106)

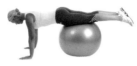

Plank
(see page 113)

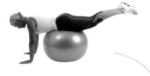

Double leg hip extension
(see page 119)

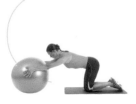

Ball roll
(see page 130)

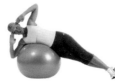

Lateral torso
flexion/extension
(see page 136)

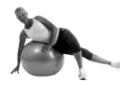

Hip adduction (ball)
(see page 141)

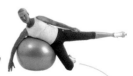

Hip abduction (ball)
(see page 139)

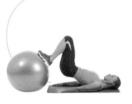

Bridge leg curl
(see page 91)

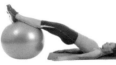

Hip extension
(see page 89)

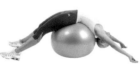

Abdominal stretch
(see page 78)

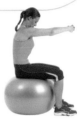

Back stretch
(see page 59)

upper body sequence

The strength and flexibility of the upper body are important in achieving and maintaining good posture and alignment. A tight chest and/or weak upper back muscles can cause rounding of the upper back (kyphosis), winging of the shoulderblades (where they stick out and lift away from the ribcage), internal rotation of the shoulders and, consequently, of the arms. Over time, this can affect a person's breathing capacity as well as the way he or she moves and carries out daily tasks.

Usually the muscles of the upper body are smaller and weaker than those of the lower body. However, as the upper body connects to the lower body, the difference in strength and flexibility between the upper and lower parts should not be so great as to result in a substantial muscular imbalance. The upper body musculature should still be able to at least lift the person's own body weight so that if we fall over or have an accident that causes us to end up on the floor, we require that upper body strength to lift our body weight to get up or to be able to crawl for help.

We ideally need a balance between the strength of the chest muscles and the strength of the upper back muscles. That commonly means that we have to stretch the chest region and strengthen the upper back.

The strength of the arms is of functional importance. If you look at the way we lift ourselves out of a chair, for example, we often use one or both arms to lever ourselves up and away from the chair. As we get older, this simple movement becomes even more important as the more mobile we remain, the better we are able to maintain an independent lifestyle.

In order to maintain functional strength in the arms we need to ensure that the biceps, triceps, shoulders and muscles of the forearms, and all the tendons and ligaments are challenged by the exercises. We also need to ensure that the joints, from the fingers through to the shoulders maintain good mobility and bone health. The following sequence will help you to achieve just that.

30–45 minutes

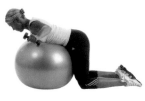

Back flye
(see page 116)

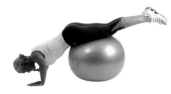

Press-up
(see page 108)

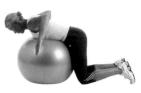

Scapula retraction
(see page 115)

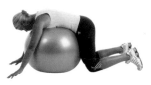

Upper back stretch
(see page 112)

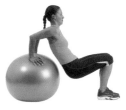

Triceps dips
(see page 69)

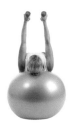

Chest flye with dumbbells
(see page 80)

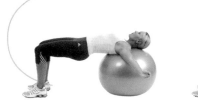

Chest stretch
(see page 77)

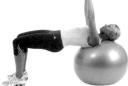

Chest press with dumbbells
(see page 81)

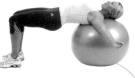

Chest stretch
(see page 77)

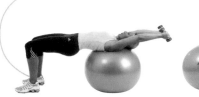

Pullover
(see page 79)

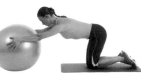

Ball roll
(see page 130)

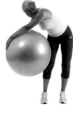

Rotary torso stretch
(see page 39)

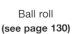

Rotator cuff
(see page 35)

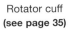

Shoulder stretch
(see page 36)

lower body sequence

Unlike the upper body, the lower body should naturally get a lot of impact movement through daily activities of standing, walking, and running. However, if someone sits for long periods of time each day, say, at their desk, in the car driving to and from work, or watching television, the lower body is not getting the demands placed on it that will keep it strong and functional.

Even if a person goes to the gym and works out for an hour but sits and/or stands relatively still for the remainder of their day, the effect of that one hour of activity will not outweigh the hours of inactivity. The reality is that in order to develop, maintain or improve general health and fitness you have to increase your overall levels of physical activity.

As with the upper body, the lower body has an important part to play in posture. Tight hip flexors will tilt the pelvis forward out of alignment and increase the curve of the lower back, adding more stress to the joints, discs, and ligaments. Tight hamstrings will tend to tilt the pelvis back so decreasing the natural curve and creating a "flat back" appearance. Tight calves can feel very uncomfortable and will affect the way you walk: these muscles need to be stretched and lengthened on a regular basis.

In many people the gluteal muscles have become lazy and the hamstrings become overactive to compensate. An indication that this is happening is when your hamstrings cramp easily or frequently. In this instance, the hamstrings need to be stretched and relaxed before a glutes exercise.

The above situation is also a reminder that stretching is not just for the end of a workout session: stretching certain muscle groups in between exercises can have a positive effect on how other, related muscles perform.

With today's sedentary lifestyles, specific lower body training is a necessity to improve and then maintain the strength and flexibility that translate into more effective and more efficient lower body movement.

30–45 minutes

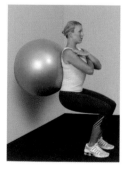 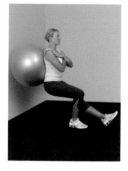 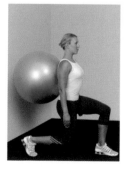 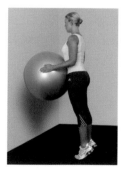

| Squat against the wall **(see page 28)** | Single leg squat against the wall **(see page 29)** | Lunge against the wall **(see page 30)** | Heel raise **(see page 31)** |

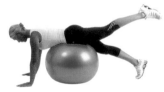

Single leg hip extension
(see page 118)

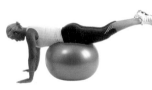

Double leg hip extension
(see page 119)

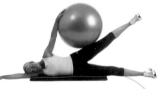

Hip abduction (floor)
(see page 138)

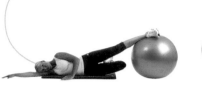

Hip adduction (floor)
(see page 140)

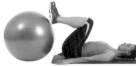

Leg curl
(see page 90)

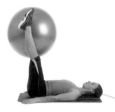

Knee extension
(see page 93)

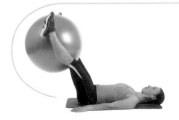

Leg press
(see page 99)

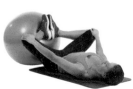

Butterfly stretch
(see page 95)

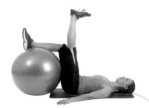

Active calf/hamstring stretch
(see page 97)

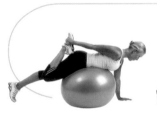

Passive quadriceps
stretch
(see page 120)

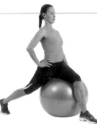

Hip flexor stretch
(see page 62)

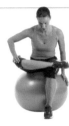

Glute stretch
(see page 67)

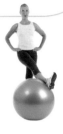

Hip abductor stretch
(see page 44)

index